MW00489458

RECOVER ALL

RECOVER ALL

A Guide for Families in Understanding Addiction

ROBERT G. REID

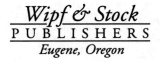

Wipf & Stock
PUBLISHERS
Eugene, Oregon

RECOVER ALL
A Guide for Families in Understanding Addiction

Copyright © 2007 Robert G. Reid. All rights reserved. Except for brief quotations in critical publications or reviews, no part of this book may be reproduced in any manner without prior written permission from the publisher. Write: Permissions, Wipf and Stock, 199 W. 8th Ave., Eugene, OR 97401.

ISBN 13: 978-1-55635-311-6

Manufactured in the U.S.A.

Scripture references marked NET [*New English Translation*] are from the NET Bible® copyright ©1996-2006 by Biblical Studies Press, L.L.C. www.bible.org All rights reserved. This material is available in its entirety as a *free download* or online web use at http://www.nextbible.org.

Scripture references marked ESV are from *The Holy Bible, English Standard Version*®, copyright © 2001 by Crossway Bibles, a publishing ministry of Good News Publishers. Used by permission. All rights reserved.

Scripture quotations marked NKJV are from *The New King James Version*®. Copyright © 1982 by Thomas Nelson, Inc. Used by permission. All rights reserved.
All emphasis in Scripture quotations have been added by the author.

The abbreviations *A.A., Alcoholics Anonymous,* and *The Big Book* are registered trademarks of Alcoholics Anonymous World Services, Inc. All Rights Reserved. (www.aa.org)

The abbreviation *N.A.* is a registered trademark of Narcotics Anonymous World Services, Inc. Reprinted by permission. All rights reserved. (www.na.org)

Throughout this work reference is made to the author's experience on staff at the House of Isaiah drug and alcohol recovery program. For more information about this program contact:

House of Isaiah—A Long-Term Drug and Alcohol Recovery Program for Men
P.O. Box 1405
Mabank, TX 75147
903-887-1373
www.HouseofIsaiah.org

Contents

Foreword

FOR THE past nineteen years I have dedicated my life to helping young men recover from drugs and alcohol. During that time I have seen thousands of young men come through my program, but I will always remember the day when this young man and his mother shared their story. I remember the desperation in his mother's voice that day as she was searching for yet another place to find help for her son. In her original call to the House of Isaiah inquiring about the program, she told the story of how many treatment centers this young man had been to, and how most recently, he had again been expelled from yet another well known program in the area. After they arrived that day, sitting at my desk with both mother and son, they described their journey. I knew there was something special about this young man. When you have worked in the field of chemical dependency as long as I have there are few stories that are really surprising. Drugs and alcohol cause people to do some really insane things, but this young man was the epitome of a hard case.

In telling their story, they described the development of a very serious heroin and cocaine addiction. Not only had his life consisted of habitual drug and alcohol abuse from a very young age, he had been to some of the most prominent treatment facilities in the country, he had seen counselors, doctors, taken medicine, and been evaluated many times. His family had spent thousands of dollars trying to get this young man the help he needed and nothing had worked. In describing the road they had traveled, I learned the treatment programs he had been to spanning four states and his extensive legal problems. Not only had he been picked up for multiple DWI's and drug charges, but also he had overdosed on heroin, an event that required paramedics to resuscitate him. If that wasn't bad enough, the director at the last treatment facility he was in told them, "He is no longer welcome in this program, and to be honest with you, I don't know of any program that can help him." It was then that I knew I wanted to work with him. I have seen the power of God transforming young men's lives through the years, and I was confident if anyone could help Rob Reid, God and the House of Isaiah program could.

In professional athletics, competition is fierce and challenges abound. One of the reasons I achieved the title NFL All-Pro Linebacker six times is because I worked hard and loved the challenge. When I founded the House of Isaiah, a long-term recovery program for men, nineteen years ago I never imagined how many "All-Pro" young men I would have the joy of helping. Nor did I recognize that day, how much God would use Rob Reid and others. I have been nothing short of amazed at his comprehension and knowledge of the disease and recovery process, his natural instinct and ability in working with families, and most of all his dedication to helping people. Rob is uniquely suited to produce this volume for families in the complex world of addiction and recovery. His lucid explanations of vital issues in recovery show his command of the subject, familiarity with the needs of families, and ability to both capture profound truths and convey them in a highly readable way. If addiction is potentially affecting someone you love, this work is indispensable. Families today, often, do not get the information they need about addiction. This has been a problem in the field of chemical dependency treatment for years. Rob saw this desperate need and has done a masterful job in addressing it. In the following pages you will learn the basics in how to navigate addiction and you will have a trustworthy guide how to—Recover All!

Isiah Robertson
House of Isaiah / Recovery Center for Men
#58 Los Angeles Rams / Buffalo Bills

Acknowledgements

MY LIFE has the great fortune of being touched by many incredible individuals, the greatest of which is Jesus Christ the Lord. In humble submission to my God, I honor my mother by dedicating this work first to her—Pat Freeman. Mom, if I know anything about love and faithfulness, I learned it from you. It was God that gave my life into your care and him that, in turn, gave you to me. Without you I would certainly have died in the grips of my drug and alcohol addiction. Thank you for never giving up—no matter what. Special thanks are due to Bill Freeman, who modeled manhood and loved me—a troubled young man—who today is grateful to be in your family.

Also, I dedicate everything valuable this work offers regarding recovery to a man who has become a father to me—Isiah Robertson. Isiah, your influence, coaching, and friendship have set my life on course to be all that God desires for me to be. I can't thank you enough, you too, never gave up on me. When no other treatment center would take me—you took me and today I have more than I could have ever dreamed. I've never known anyone as committed to serving the Lord at any cost, thank you for all you do and the thousands you have and continue to help.

Additionally, I thank my wife—Christine—whose love I cherish, Micam, the son who is as my own, and to Gennavieve my daughter. Without your prayers, encouragement, and love I couldn't have brought this work to completion. You, Micam, and Genna make our home and family an incredible adventure. Thanks also to Chet, Sue, Beth, Jeff, Jamie, Bonnie, Don, Jason, and Brea—for your love and support.

To my father Bill Reid and Ginger, thank you both for your kind words and encouragement. Thank you to my grandmother Betty Sterry who always said I would write and James Sterry Sr. for all you taught me. Thanks to W. L. and Margaret Reid, truly grandparents who have modeled what it is to love and serve the Lord—thank you for all your support through the years.

Finally, I want to honor the people who poured into my life, some realized their influence more than others, but today my spiritual life and love for studying God's Word and indeed, my character, was and continues to be largely shaped by these to whom I am very grateful: Professors Daniel B. Wallace, Paul Alexander, Bruce Rosdahl, Joseph Fantin, Darryl Bock, and

Richard Hanner. My prayer is that God might allow me to teach with the same faithfulness, tireless dedication, and love which you each have modeled for me. Thanks are due also to the following pastors for their influence, support, and help in following God's calling on my life: Barry Boatright, Bob Nichols, Kenny White, and most recently Ron Holton. Also, the following teachers believed in me during my teenage years, when no one else did: Mary Conrad, Sally Teeman, Larry Bonk, Tim Lashombe, and Ona Winders. Last, but certainly not least, I thank the community of faithful friends who deserve credit for seeing me through my own development in this enterprise we call life: Reuben Olivarez, David Hoinides, Dallas Gingles, John Heifner, Tim Taylor, Charles Banno, Tryston Gordy, and James Salinas.

Thanks are also due to Wipf and Stock publishing, and especially Jim Tedrick and Carrie Wolcott for helping to bring this project to realization.

Introduction

SEARCHING FOR answers about addiction can be a very grueling task. Amidst the many voices of assistance available, few seem to offer the simple and practical help that is needed—then comes the arduous undertaking of attempting to sift through the psychobabble and medical documentation. All this is done in hopes of finding some useful answers for a real problem. Where are the authentic people who have been where I am? Can anyone just give me some *real* guidance? It wasn't long ago that my own family was wondering these same things. They battled for over ten years to save my life from my perilous addiction. Seldom did they ever receive the direct, practical support and advice they needed. My mother scoured scores of books seeking answers in order to help her try to keep her drug-addicted son alive. These books were full of wonderful advice for people. The authors were reputable doctors, psychiatrists, and counselors who had spent years studying addiction. The only problem was that they didn't really *know* addiction. They had countless classroom hours studying addiction theory, but outside of clinical theories and principles they hadn't really experienced the condition they were treating. It is for this reason that this work is different.

Recover All: A Guide for Families in Understanding Addiction is written specifically for you. It's not a medical journal or clinical review. The sole purpose of its content is to share the experience, strength, and hope of recovery so that you, the family, can understand it. Within its pages you will find a simple overview of addiction and the addictive process. It is intended to provide practical education that will empower your family to succeed in recovery.

Even if you're not sure if your loved one has an addiction here you will find substantial evidence in helping to identify whether or not addiction is a concern in your circumstances. Real life stories of addicts and their families will warm your heart and guard you against their mistakes. So now you're wondering, who is the author? What qualifies him to be a reliable voice about addiction? I have spent more than half of my life as an addict of various drugs. Clinically, my case was diagnosed as poly-substance abuse. Principally, in rudimentary terms "Poly-Substance

Abuser" boils down to: if a drug would get you high, I would do it. A poly-substance abuser is an individual who uses many different classes of substances indiscriminately without having a specific drug that qualifies for dependence. Over the course of my addiction, I've attended multiple treatment programs in excess of nine times, seen the foremost addiction-ologists in the South, and experienced virtually every mainstream form of drug treatment available.

After successfully recovering from active daily addiction, I worked on staff at the House of Isaiah, a long-term drug and alcohol treatment center for men. While on faculty, the experience of working with addicts, their families, and the treatment staff fashioned a great deal of my own thinking pertaining to addiction, the addictive process, and recovery. With half-a-lifetime of experience being the addict and manipulating my own family, I learned how to effectively help addicts and their families in the healing process. Thus, I understand what it is to sit on both sides of the treatment dynamic, namely, as the addict and as the case manager and administrator. Having spent so much of my life's focus dealing with addiction and work-ing with other families in the same situation, I believe that what I have to share with you subsequently will benefit your family in immeasurable ways and equip you to navigate the frigid and terrifying waters of addic-tion without experiencing the same pitfalls many other family members have struggled through.

Since getting clean and sober, my life has been dedicated to helping other people overcome addiction. It is my passion to educate families of the warning signs and behaviors that they need to be aware of. Through my experience, I found a serious disjunction between chemical dependen-cy treatment for the individual and the family (family being used broadly for anyone associated with the addict's life personally). While most of the patients were receiving qualitatively and quantitatively useful information about recovery, their family was left in the dark, as it were. The few av-enues which address the family and loved ones of the addict often failed to meet their needs, that is, their questions, problems, and information pertinent to what they experience as a result of their loved one's addic-tion (and treatment process). In response to this, *Recover All: A Guide for Families in Understanding Addiction* sets a new paradigm. The family now has a voice of hope and channel of counsel.

1

What Is Addiction?

ADDICTION IS by far one of the most elusive topics within the realm of human thought. This is resultant of it being a study of human behavior and thereby a study of human thinking as it relates to behavior. Though most dismiss its importance, those who find themselves in its maddening grip ever grapple for sufficient knowledge and help apprehending the subject matter. Below, we will attempt to assimilate an, albeit "rough," working understanding of addiction, for a family member unversed in psychological, clinical rhetoric. Our hope is that virtually anyone's understanding of addiction would be significantly furthered by reading this section.

In the course of what follows, two terms will be used: alcoholism and addiction. There is great overlap in the meaning of these terms, as well as variation, since they are not identical. Properly, addiction is a broader categorical term, which refers to a compulsive behavior involving some substance or explicit behavior. That is, addiction can involve one of virtually any "substances" (i.e., food, nicotine, heroin, sex, etc.). Alcoholism refers to addiction, but is much more precise in that it describes addiction *to* (or at least involving) *alcohol.* Therefore, alcoholism is a subset category of the more inclusive (and less precise) term: addiction. In the final analysis, however, the terms for our present concern may be held as virtually synonymous. For instance, the phenomenon of alcoholism, pertaining to an individual's use of alcohol is fundamentally identical to the phenomenon of heroin addiction, with the only difference being the substance. Thus, when we speak of *alcoholism* and *addiction* we are referring to the mental and behavioral relationship of the human to the "substance" (whether that substance is heroin, alcohol, sex, etc.). Thus, the terms "addiction" and "alcoholism" will be used interchangeably throughout this work. Offering some further insight concerning alcoholism, the Alcoholics Anonymous program's *The Big Book*® gives great clarity in understanding alcoholism/addiction. We will consult this work several times to help give shape to our topic. Thus, we ask again, "What is addiction/alcoholism?" In order

3

to articulate anything one must begin somewhere or with a first question; hence, we ask, "*who* are alcoholics and addicts?"

> The classification of alcoholics seems most difficult . . . There are of course, the psychopaths who are emotionally unstable. We are familiar with this type. They are over-remorseful and make many resolutions, but never a decision. There is a type of man who is unwilling to admit that he cannot take a drink. He plans various ways of drinking. He changes his brand or his environment. There is the type who always believes that after being entirely free from alcohol for a period of time he can take a drink without danger. There is the manic-depressive type, who is perhaps, the least understood by his friends, and about whom a whole chapter could be written. Then there are types entirely normal in every respect except in the effect alcohol has upon them. They are often able, intelligent, friendly people. All these, and many others, have one symptom in common: they cannot start drinking without developing the phenomenon of craving. This phenomenon, as we have suggested, may be the manifestation of an allergy, which differentiates these people, and sets them apart as a distinct entity. It has never been, by any treatment with which we are familiar, permanently eradicated. The only relief we have to suggest is entire abstinence.[1]

As you can see the manifestation of alcoholism and addiction can be seen in a variety of forms. It is no respecter of persons. Addiction affects all levels of education, economic status, race, color, and creed. In order to properly frame the issue of addiction, all those preconceived ideas that have been fostered through your life experience must be evaluated, and in some sense, set aside. At least, we must re-evaluate what an "addict" looks like, practically speaking.

When one imagines an "addict" or "alcoholic" they typically picture a street person, one poor, dirty, and alone in the world. The irony of our deluded mental images of the addict on the street is the reality that most addicts are educated, have families, hold down jobs, etc. Some of them are executives of major corporations. For instance, it is entirely possible that your accountant or the nurse who took your blood pressure at your last doctor's visit might have been an addict. Addiction, generally speaking, is a phenomenon predominately fostered in middle to upper-middle class economies. I grew up thinking addiction and alcoholism were safely confined under the bridge or in low-income communities, but that simply

---

1. William D. Silkworth, "The Doctor's Opinion," in *Alcoholics Anonymous*, xxviii.

is not the case. We would do well to keep our eyes wide open to the possibility and probability of addiction being within, even our own family.

It is important to note that *not every person* who uses drugs or alcohol will become an addict or alcoholic. This is usually one of the greatest hindrances to parents being able to perceive their child's addictive behavior. For instance, when warning signs of possible chemical abuse arise, the typical parent will simply attribute or correlate that behavior with some of their own experimentation with drugs or alcohol in high school or college. They calm their apprehension by telling themselves, "Everyone goes through *that phase.*" However, *that* is not the case. There are multitudes of people who, once they begin drinking or using, *lose all control*—these are real alcoholics/addicts. We find the most illuminating illustration of this on page 21 of *Alcoholics Anonymous*:

> Here is the fellow who has been puzzling you, especially in his lack of control. He does absurd, incredible, tragic things while drinking. He is a real Dr. Jekyll and Mr. Hyde. He is seldom mildly intoxicated. He is always more or less insanely drunk. His disposition while drinking resembles his normal nature but little. He may be one of the finest fellows in the world. Yet let him drink for a day, and he frequently becomes disgustingly, and even dangerously anti-social. He has a positive genius for getting tight at exactly the wrong moment, particularly when some important decision must be made or engagement kept. He is often perfectly sensible and well balanced concerning everything except liquor, but in that respect he is incredibly dishonest and selfish. He often possesses special abilities, skills, and aptitudes, and has a promising career ahead of him. He uses his gifts to build up a bright outlook for his family and himself, and then pulls the structure down on his head by a senseless series of sprees. He is the fellow who goes to bed so intoxicated he ought to sleep the clock around. Yet early next morning he searches madly for the bottle he misplaced the night before. If he can afford it, he may have liquor concealed all over his house to be certain no one gets his entire supply away from him to throw down the wastepipe. As matters grow worse, he begins to use a combination of high-powered sedative and liquor to quiet his nerves so he can go to work. Then comes the day when he simply cannot make it and gets drunk all over again.[2]

If this description seems all too familiar, whether the substance is alcohol or drugs, you are reading the right material. This is a pristine picture of what alcoholism/addiction looks like to the family and friends.

2. *Alcoholics Anonymous*, 22.

Certainly, it is not a comprehensive picture, but should provide a rough sketch to anyone of the characteristics of an addict/alcoholic. Addiction/alcoholism is accepted today in the medical community as a disease. The disease concept of addiction/alcoholism, as Dr. Silkworth so wonderfully pioneered, is comprised of two parts *the mental obsession coupled with a physical allergy.* The mental obsession or "phenomenon of craving" is the drive that usurps importance in the mind of the addict/alcoholic to consume more of the chemical. The mental obsession aspect could very well be the most obscure facet of the disease. This phenomenon of craving compels the addict/alcoholic to consume more of the chemical. It also includes the thought processes that delude the individual's ability to realize the problem.

The "physical allergy" is the adverse reaction experienced in the body of the addict when the chemical is consumed. To make this model easier, think of it like an allergy to penicillin. If a person were allergic to penicillin, when the drug was ingested that person would experience a reaction. The reaction could be a rash, hives, vomiting, or a number of other adverse consequences. The physical body of the alcohol/addict has an undesirable reaction in the same way. A somewhat more amusing way to think of it can be illustrated in the following statement: "People who are allergic to penicillin break out in hives, when an alcoholic/addict drinks/drugs they break out in hand-cuffs." Alcohol and drugs cause a reaction, one of genuine insanity, in the addict's decision making processes and set in motion the mental obsession to consume more. There is presently no medical cure for addiction/alcoholism. The only solution is abstinence. To the addict, who typically thinks in terms of quick fixes, this diagnosis seems completely untenable. However, for the addict, abstinence is not a matter of self-will. If self-will could stop the supposed addict/alcoholic for any *extended period* of time, it is likely that the person in question might not be "alcoholic/addicted." So the only viable solution for those who are truly chemically dependent is to participate in a program of recovery.

Abstinence is achieved for the addict/alcoholic by working a program. "Working a program" means doing those things which are necessary to keep from using chemicals on a daily basis. This includes (but is not limited to): attending Alcoholics Anonymous/Narcotics Anonymous meetings (abbreviated A.A./N.A., respectively), working the steps, working with a sponsor, being involved in church, praying, *et cetera.* So what is addiction? Addiction is a perplexing malady. I have known many spiritual leaders who would deny that alcoholism/addiction is a disease, but most that hold this view are limited in their experience with addicts and knowledge of addiction. That is to say, when an individual hasn't experienced working one-on-one with an addicted person it is easy for him or her to develop many misconceptions, the most common of which is merely to attribute addiction to a lack of discipline or self-control. In my own life, there were both family members and friends who thought that above all my chief problems were ones of will power and poor decision making.

As you read this page, you might be thinking along those same lines. We all begin to come to terms with addiction first from our preconceived ideas and then we work from there, but I challenge you to think through the possibility that addiction is a disease, in some ways like cancer, but in other ways completely different. Indeed, if someone were to ask me to give an analogy or ask what I would relate addiction to, at least categorically in terms of illness or disease, I think it is most closely related to a mental illness such as bi-polar or schizophrenia. Granted there are vast differences and these are merely analogies, the point is that addiction bears with it two aspects, namely, an aspect of responsibility for ones own decisions and mental choices, but it also incorporates the other aspect somewhat in tension with the former—that is, mental and biological factors that are completely outside the control of the addict (i.e., heredity and possibly other factors). Through much pain and misery I have come to the conclusion that addiction is a disease. And yet, classifying addiction as a disease doesn't make alcoholics or addicts irresponsible for their use. The disease concept is not to be used as a crutch or justification. People who are addicted/alcoholic do not necessarily need to be treated as disabled persons or with a special temperament, exclusively on the basis of addiction. As with anyone with a mental illness, the addict is responsible to take the steps necessary to treat their disease and go about living a productive life.

Just like a cancer patient, addicts must actively participate in their treatment, however painful that may be at times. The interesting thing about addiction is the mental illusion. What we mean here is that most cancer patients (once diagnosed) do not *tell* themselves that they *do not* really have cancer. Usually, they don't stop taking the medicine or chemotherapy prescribed to them based on their own opinion that they really are not sick (unless, of course, they have some type of death wish). Addicts on the other hand do just that. Addiction is one of the only diseases that in mental "talk" tells the addict they don't really have the disease. The expression of this is characterized in the first text we cited, stating:

> There is a type of man who is unwilling to admit that he cannot take a drink. He plans various ways of drinking. He changes his brand or his environment. There is the type who always believes

that after being entirely free from alcohol for a period of time he can take a drink without danger.[3]

This is the most startling and strange manifestation of addiction. It doesn't make sense to the common mind. Why would anyone deny the truth or be so blind to all the signs? This has perplexed many throughout history. Rather than attempting to "solve" the conundrum, we must acknowledge and be practically aware that a characteristic of addiction is the unwillingness to admit—an inability to drink or use like "normal" people.

Notice in the text above how the same man who is unwilling to admit that he cannot drink also goes to great lengths to plan various attempts to do just that, namely, to drink normally. Addicts persist in attempting to "out wit" their addiction. In an attempt to give further clarity to the portrait of addiction, let us look at another example. We suggest, this type of person exhibits in action, what is by definition: alcoholic/addicted *insanity*. Indeed, a lucid demonstration of this is articulated in the following:

> Most of us have been unwilling to admit we were real alcoholics. No person likes to think he is bodily and mentally different from his fellows. Therefore, it is not surprising that our drinking careers have been characterized by countless vain attempts to prove we could drink like other people. *The idea that somehow, someday he will control and enjoy his drinking is the great obsession of every abnormal drinker.* The persistence of this illusion is astonishing. Many pursue it into the gates of insanity or death. We learned that we had to fully concede to our innermost selves that we were alcoholics. This is the first step in recovery. The delusion that we are like other people, or presently may be, has to be smashed. We alcoholics are men and women who have lost the ability to control our drinking. We know that no real alcoholic *ever* recovers control. All of us felt at times that we were regaining control, but such intervals-usually brief-were inevitably followed by still less control, which led in time to pitiful and incomprehensible demoralization. We are convinced to a man that alcoholics of our type are in the grip of a progressive illness. Over any considerable period we get worse, never better. We are like men who have lost their legs; they never grow new ones. Neither does there appear to be any kind of treatment, which will make alcoholics of our kind like other men. We have tried every imaginable remedy. In some instances there has been brief recovery, followed always by a still worse relapse. Physicians who are familiar with alcoholism agree there is no such

3. Silkworth, xxviii.

thing as making a normal drinker out of an alcoholic. Science may one day accomplish this, but it hasn't done so yet. Despite all we can say, many who are real alcoholics are not going to believe they are in that class. By every form of self-deception and experimentation, they will try to prove themselves exceptions to the rule, therefore nonalcoholic . . . Here are some of the methods we have tried: Drinking beer only, limiting the number of drinks, never drinking alone, never drinking in the morning, drinking only at home, never having it in the house, never drinking during business hours, drinking only at parties, switching from scotch to brandy, drinking only natural wines, agreeing to resign if ever drunk on the job, taking a trip, not taking a trip, swearing off forever (with and without a solemn oath), taking more physical exercise, reading inspirational books, going to health farms and sanitariums, accepting voluntary commitment to asylums-we could increase the list ad infinitum.[4]

This text captures the very essence of the issue of addicted/alcoholic insanity. People who are truly addicted never want to admit it or accept it. To accept it would mean to face the reality of an existing *problem* and be forced, in some sense, to address it and *change*. To change means to stop using, and for an addict that is not an option. The persistence of the illusion that one can drink or use like "normal" people has led to the deaths of many. Until one resolves that he or she is in fact alcoholic/addicted, they cannot begin the process of recovery. This condition of addiction is irreversible, meaning that *no matter* how long a person stays clean and sober, the addiction will spring back in full force if chemicals are ingested. It is so important that you, the family of the addict, understand this is not merely *a phase*, if you are genuinely dealing with addiction. Your loved one, if a true addict/alcoholic, will not be able to have a glass of wine with dinner, or just smoke one joint on a holiday. *Ever!*

To believe that would be utter deception, in so far as, by definition an addict is unable to use without the mental obsession and physical allergy rising to prominence again. In my experience working with families, unfortunately, they notoriously misunderstand this very aspect of addiction, that abstinence for a period of time does not offset the mental obsession or physical allergy anymore than a person who is deathly allergic to peanuts, after a year or two, should be able to eat a peanut safely. The hardest thing for treatment personnel to do (other than dealing with the individual addicts) is communicate this understanding concerning addiction

4. *Alcoholics Anonymous*, 30, emphasis added.

to the family—recovery requires a *permanent* change of lifestyle. Wine with dinner or social drinking/using will never be an option. *For if the addict/alcoholic does use, even just once, they will have unleashed the monster of addiction as if it had never left.*

Addiction is a progressive illness. It progressively gets worse. Even when drugs and alcohol are not used, the addiction, even in remission, is at all times potentially as terrible as before. In fact, many cases I have seen of relapse appear as though the addiction worsened though chemicals were not used. Thus, though a person abstain from drinking and drugs for a time, it would be irresponsible to think that their addiction had decreased in intensity if they were to use again. Many who have achieved any notable sobriety (only to relapse) find out all to well that the severity of their addiction had progressed significantly, though they did not use chemicals.

From this it is reasonable to gather also that addiction is oftentimes a system of coping. Many people develop chemical dependencies (note that some develop *a* chemical dependency, while in my case I developed many chemical dependencies) resultant from fleeing emotionally from other issues. For instance: to self-medicate from depression people will turn to chemicals or drugs. Perhaps to run from insecurity, one will turn to drinking in order to have confidence at social gatherings. More will be said about this in later sections, but for the present purposes it is helpful to understand that people frequently develop addiction over time and there are always other pertinent circumstances, which is to say, there are a variety of factors and influences to the development and perpetuation of addiction, all of which deserve to be taken into consideration.

Now the question comes to mind for the Christian: "Isn't it possible for God to deliver my loved one from addiction?" The answer is simple: yes. God, however, at least in light of biblical revelation and Christian history does not appear to be in the business of being a "divine enabler." If you find yourself thinking along these lines, notice that the question fundamentally presupposes, what in the present author's opinion is a *skewed* perspective of what deliverance by definition is. When God delivers someone from the grips of addiction that does not mean that the delivered person can drink socially without recourse or regression to past alcoholic/addicted tendencies. It simply does not follow that God would deliver his children out of "Egypt" in order for them to be able to participate in Egyptian cultural practices, the likes of which God does not endorse. Why be delivered from imprisonment only to return to "hang out" with your former captors? Furthermore, as a Christian minister myself, I am very hesitant to merely punt to deliverance. I firmly believe that God has delivered me from my addiction; however, at the same time I firmly believe that while he did the work in changing my heart, I had to do the work in learning how to live and practice a life in sobriety. Therefore, I am very leery of approaches to treat addiction that are exclusive in the sense that the *only* means to healing and recovery is found in prayer and Bible reading. My experience has been that a *holistic* approach is the best, namely, one that addresses cognitive and behavioral aspects of the individual (i.e., counseling, chemical dependency education, group counseling, etc.) along with a genuinely Christian aspect (Bible study, education, counseling, etc.).

We conclude then, that alcoholism/addiction is a disease. It is also a spiritual malady. Both of these dialectical distinctives are significant and neither can be left out of the equation. Thus, addiction is both a disease (mental obsession coupled with a physical allergy) and a spiritual malady. The only way to win is to surrender, a principle fundamentally at odds with common sense, ego, and self-will. Our somewhat flexible definition is as follows: addiction is a harmful, abnormal human condition (or *state of living*) that is multi-dimensional in scope, namely, physiological, neurological, and spiritual that manifests in relation to dependence upon a substance (whether physical or behavioral [as stated above]) and produces negative life consequences for the individual addict and those around him or her. Therefore, addiction is the *condition* underlying the outward negative effects of human dependence upon a substance. This section will close with a passage that radically influenced my life, because it spoke directly to my condition and hopefully will speak to your circumstance and understanding as well. May it bless you and help you to understand addiction:

> For most normal folks, drinking means conviviality, companionship and colorful imagination. It means release from care, boredom and worry. It is joyous intimacy with friends and a feeling that life is good. But not so with us in those last days of heavy drinking. The old pleasures were gone. They were but memories. Never could we recapture the great moments of the past. There was an insistent yearning to enjoy life as we once did and a heartbreaking obsession that some new miracle of control would enable us to do it. There was always one more attempt and one more failure. The less people tolerated us, the more we withdrew from society, from life itself. As we became subjects of King Alcohol, shivering denizens of his mad realm, the chilling vapor that is loneliness settled down. It thickened, ever becoming blacker. Some of us sought out sordid places, hoping to find understanding companionship and approval. Momentarily we did—then would come oblivion and the awful awakening to face the hideous Four Horsemen—Terror,

Bewilderment, Frustration, Despair. Unhappy drinkers who read this page will understand! Now and then a serious drinker, being dry at the moment says, "I don't miss it at all. Feel better. Work better. Having a better time." As ex-problem drinkers we smile at such a sally. We know our friend is like a boy whistling in the dark to keep up his spirits. He fools himself. Inwardly he would give anything to take half a dozen drinks and get away with them. He will presently try the old game again, for he isn't happy about his sobriety. He cannot picture life without alcohol. Some day he will be unable to imagine either life with alcohol or with out it. Then he will know loneliness such as few do. He will be at the jumping off place. He will wish for the end.[5]

5. *Alcoholics Anonymous*, 152, emphasis added.

2

How Addiction Develops

IT CAN be a very perplexing thing to attempt to understand how your loved one developed addiction. To many it seems somewhat mysterious. There are those who assert that it was genetic. Others demand it was the influence of wicked spiritual forces. In reality, we simply do not know with any certainty. Therefore, it is possible that the answer is not either/or, but rather both/and. Thus, taking into account our present definition as described in the previous chapter that addiction is multi-dimensional, that is, physiological, neurological, and spiritual, then we conclude the answer is: all of the above. We return then to the logical question: how did our loved one develop an addiction?

From the information gleaned in the previous chapter, it may be becoming more obvious to you now that addiction is probable in regards to your loved one. The question in your mind though, is how? How did this happen? When did it all start? Addiction tends to take the family by surprise. For so long addicted persons are able to appear as if everything is copasetic. However, inwardly things are worse than they have ever been. So together we will seek to answer these questions in a down to earth and practical manner that anyone can understand.

The Reward Center

At the very mention of the word "reward," people's eyebrows tend to raise in anticipation. Everyone likes rewards. Visa and MasterCard multiply their customer base each year offering "incentive and reward" programs. People love to be rewarded. After mowing your lawn or tending to the responsibilities of your home, you sit back on your couch and "reward" yourself with a chocolate sundae and a nap. It is not hard for us to grasp the concept of *reward*. Even your dog understands the reward system. In fact, that's how humans typically train animals.

It goes something like this: "Rover lay down! Good Boy." Then you hand him a doggy treat. Once the dog learns how the system works, his entire behavior pattern adjusts to accommodate the new reward system. When I was a young child we had a small Shitzu dog. His name was Peanut. He loved cheese. So in an attempt to train Peanut to sit, we used a reward system based on cheese. Each time he would obey the command, he would be rewarded. If he did not do the action requested, he was not rewarded. In the midst of this, however, Peanut displayed an interesting adaptation to the learned behavior. Not only did he learn to sit, but he also attempted to manipulate this cause/effect relationship in such a way that he could initiate the cause. He began doing the behavior "sitting" in order to *get* the desired result, rather than when the master commanded. Therefore, he short-circuited his learned behavior because he stopped doing the "sitting" on command. He had deduced that the act of sitting got him a pleasurable reward.

The human brain has a unique system of rewards as well. There is actually an area of the brain known medically as the "reward center" (part of the limbic system) of the brain. This is the area where neurotransmitters fire between the receptor cells in the brain. For instance, when a woman experiences an orgasm sexually, there is a chemical released in the brain that produces immense pleasure. The male's body functions identically regarding the reward center. When a runner runs a great distance and experiences a "runner's high," this is really just a chemical release in the reward center of their brain. Every pleasure we have in life results from certain neurotransmitters creating a "pathway" where specific hormones and cerebral chemicals are released—causing the reward feeling.

Ivan Pavlov a well-known psychiatrist deduced from these findings what I call the "ring the bell, feed the dog, ring the bell, spank the dog" theory (or formally "classical conditioning"). It is an understanding of the way the brain can be trained. If a bell is rung consistently when your dog is being fed, within a short time the dog will have *associated* the bell with the food. This means that now, thirty days later you can ring the bell and the dog's mouth begins to salivate. He runs over to his food bowl expecting food to be there. Conversely, the opposite can happen if every time you discipline your dog you ring a bell. He associates the bell with the discipline. So thirty days or so later when he hears the bell, he immediately cowers in fear. He expects discipline and thinks he has done something wrong. Why? He associates the sound with the effect.

Let's look at this now from another perspective. For the pornography addict this same principle holds true. Most pornography addicts are addicted to masturbation. When they climax, the chemical in the brain is released. Each time their brain releases that chemical what is in front of their eyes? Pornography, of course. So what do you think their brain associates? The pictures of nudity are associated with the chemical release of climax. It is for this reason that pornography destroys marriage. The husband who views pornography is subconsciously linked to the pictures instead of his wife. So, many times during sexual relations, he will find himself imagining the women from the pornography he has viewed. The reason is because his brain has correlated the pictures and the chemical release, instead of with his wife.

In the case of the drug addict the same scenario plays out. Each time the crack addict sees a certain sign on the highway, his stomach gets tight and his palms sweat in anticipation. The reason is because every time he takes that exit, he buys and uses crack. So his brain has developed a pathway. The brain is fully aware that it will receive the reward if the action is taken. Therefore, it begins preparing itself for euphoria. This manifests in anxiousness, sweaty palms, imagining the high, etc.

It is vital that you understand that regardless of addiction or alcoholism, every human brain, including yours, functions in this way. You have the same reward system. Your brain correlates specific activities with pleasure. For you it may be a cigarette first thing in the morning. It could be the feeling of a job well done. Regardless of what it is, you are no different, all humanity shares in these behavioral qualities. All humanity participates in association of behaviors and neurological chemical releases in the brain.

We must keep this in mind if we are ever to form a comprehensive understanding of addiction and how it develops. All addicts, no matter the type (food, sex, drugs, shopping, etc.) essentially are "drug addicts." They are addicted to the release of chemicals in their brain. These are learned behaviors. Once a pathway is developed it never goes away. The addict can't have the "pathway" removed when it becomes unpleasant. The only effective way to deal with these pathways is to "unlearn" the behavior. This essentially means *retraining* the brain. Once I attended a conference, primarily geared towards ministry to sex addicts. While there I was introduced to one means of assisting the sex addict in realigning their thought patterns or re-training their brain.

One method suggested at the conference involved re-training the brain by using a rubber band. Now, of course, this was geared towards lust and sexual addiction, but it could be used for anything. The idea was this. The patient would wear a rubber band on their wrist. Just like a bracelet. Each time that person started to stare at a woman and lust they were instructed to "pop" the rubber band against their wrist. That hurts! That is exactly the point. Over about a thirty-day period, the brain will begin to associate looking lustfully at a woman with that pain. Ring the bell, spank the dog. The whole concept effectively takes what has been a pleasure and retrains the brain to associate it with pain. Thus, the individual's behavior has been modified. This is really a brilliant tool. It may sound slightly rudimentary, but I have seen it work in some of my client's lives!

The Progressive Phases of the Development of Addiction

Addiction is not a "fly-by-night" disorder. Though it startles most and takes them by surprise, it does not develop overnight. It starts small and progresses, ever growing in a snowball effect. Then before most see it coming, it overwhelms them. Cancer and addiction are very similar to think about. Cancer starts from one cell—just one little, tiny microscopic cell. Cells reproduce themselves. Cancer originates with a single cell that mutates. The mutation occurs during the reproduction process by a slight variation. That variation produces a cell that is *not* a replica of the original. The DNA of the cell is perverted from the original leaving a mutation. Then, day-by-day, that cell multiplies.

As the cell multiplies, it obviously reproduces cells like itself, only mutated. These cells continue to multiply exponentially causing a mass to form. The mass continues to grow. If the cancer mass or tumor isn't detected, it can possibly begin to travel through the lymphatic system around the body. As it travels, it produces its mutated cells around the body. If the cancer goes undetected for too long, it passes our ability to effectively treat it. There is presently no cure for cancer. The only help for those who develop it is early detection. Addiction/alcoholism is virtually identical in this regard. There is no cure. The only hope is early detection and treatment. Some cancer patients have the mass(es) removed and undergo extensive chemical therapy. Some live and make it the rest of their lives cancer-free. Others, sadly, do not. Sometimes treatment doesn't work for everyone. Then we have little explanation other than we just should have caught it sooner.

Addiction develops as one thought or system of thought that becomes perverted. It grows and grows. If undetected it (like cancer) is eventually terminal. It can develop for years before it's ever noticed. Then suddenly, during a routine exam, it is revealed! How did this happen? When did it start? Why me? There are five phases in the development of addiction. Each of these phases represents an undefined period of time. For some it may be days, while for others it may be years or decades. Each phase has distinctive characteristics and builds upon the previous. These phases are progressive.

The five phases of addiction are:

Phase One: Infatuation
Phase Two: The Love Affair
Phase Three: Infidelity
Phase Four: Great Distress
Phase Five: Imprisoned

Five Phases
Phase One: Infatuation

The first phase encompasses the great days of pleasure. These are the first days of chemical use. During this time the initial love is spawned. There is newness with the chemical, much in the same way that new relationships develop between men and women. The first time they meet there is attraction and suspense. Newly dating couples often are filled with wonder and amazement. Each time they meet they learn more about each other. They exchange those first looks and first kisses. This phase is a time in which the person exchanges the "firsts" with their drug of choice. They are filled with wonder, imaging all the future, wonderful times they can foresee in their mind's eye.

During this phase, the person will look to the chemical(s) as attractive lovers. They will seem to be in a "starry-eyed" infatuation. It is during this time when they are simply amazed at the chemical's ability to make them feel so wonderful. They will be fascinated with the lifestyle.

This is the time that the neuro-pathway originates. The bell has rung and the reward has been handed out. These are the memories which this person will hold dear throughout the course of the addictive process. Now the brain is fully aware of the pleasure the drug has to offer. The imprint on the mind has been made. Infatuation has begun.

Phase Two: The Love Affair

These are the early days of the beginning addiction. Using is still fun. A good analogy or way to think about this is as a love affair. Extra-marital affairs begin with infatuation. Then the affair takes place. Rarely is real "love" ever developed, but the affair is an attempt to recapture the "first" love from the infatuation phase. The duration of the love affair can vary per the individual. During it the "lustful desires" are rewarded. This is true in the case of the developing addict. This is the season where using is fulfilling the need. It is still serving its purpose. So if the person in question is running from fear, guilt, shame, or any other feeling during this phase, the chemical is actually temporarily satisfying that concern.

During this phase, the addictive person learns that the drug "works" to fix the problem. Once the issue has been seemingly "fixed" or suppressed, namely, the undesirable feeling(s), the mind of the addict perceives this as having accomplished the goal. You must realize that there was a time in the addicted person's developing addiction when the drug or drink actually did work for the purpose they desired. It really did alleviate the emotional pain momentarily. When this happened, the love affair was in full swing. The chemical now has proved its ability to ease the pain. Thus, the addictive person has learned to *depend* on the chemical for satisfaction. During this phase, using was "working," so to speak, for the addict.

Phase Three: Infidelity

Phase three is treachery in regard to the relationship between the person and the chemical. The hideous horseman has inflicted his wounding blow. During this process something gets "broken" in the series of behaviors and their expected outcomes. No one really knows what day or hour this metaphorical line is crossed. Once, however, this line of demarcation has been crossed it may never be revisited. This is a major landmark on the road towards full-blown addiction. The reason for this conclusion lies in the fact that the chemical betrays the user. Suddenly, the chemicals are no longer having the effect that they once were. That is, the addict begins developing tolerance to the chemical. Tolerance, however, is not limited to physical tolerance, of which a few words must be said. First, physical tolerance occurs when the quantitative amount of the user's drug of choice no longer brings the same qualitative effect.

Another way to think about this would be to imagine an alcoholic. Initially, he might get completely drunk from 6 to 8 shots of whiskey, whereas that same individual only one year later, after having consumed whiskey frequently on the weekends throughout that year, may have developed enough tolerance to the alcohol that it may take significantly more shots to produce the same drunken effect. Thus, this is physical tolerance, but there are other aspects of tolerance which are pertinent to the discussion—namely, emotional tolerance. This is evidenced in the individual who employs the use of their drug of choice for the purpose of suppressing or temporarily forgetting their problems. Once the pattern is developed of "covering" one's negative feelings with chemicals, addicts typically find more and more "feelings" that need to be suppressed. This is slightly more difficult to articulate, but for the sake of illustration, let's say John uses alcohol to cover up insecurity and feel confident. After practicing this type of self-medication in the area of insecurity, with some desired effect, John is prone to begin self-medicating in other areas also. During this process the chemical becomes less effective to the specific area addressed, that is, the addict develops emotional tolerance in the sense that it requires more of the chemical to be "happy" or "at peace." Eventually, the emotional pain is no longer being alleviated. No longer are troubles being forgotten in the daze of chemical euphoria. Something has broken!

During this phase, the insanity of addiction ensues. The addict is now growing desperate. That thing which has been soothing their anxieties and providing them with pleasure has failed to meet their need. The great affair of yesterday has fizzled out today, as most do. For the reason that: infatuation never was love. The affair was merely indulgence and now the initial excitement has worn off. Suddenly, the seductress is purely a conquered land, which offers no stimulation. Therefore, the addict wields the learned instrument of personal chemical therapy for quantitatively more emotional support and/or relief and the effectuality of such a release, decreases.

Phase Four: Great Distress

To some, the names of these phases might at first glance seem to be overstated, though I think, from the addict's perspective these phases are just as dramatic as their titles imply. The "great distress" ensues as the next logical outworking of the digression which began in the previous phase. Desperately, the addict uses more and more in hopes of revisiting past pleasures. Each attempt unlocks the door to even greater disappointment. Now the addict begins to feel like an individual used purely for sexual fulfillment—empty, used, and alone.

During this phase, the addictive insanity flourishes. Day after day, weekend after weekend, they practice the same behavior of ingesting chemicals, which by this point have ceased producing the desired results, yet the addict expects "this time" to be different. They use, never achieving the high or the escape they hoped for. Then madly they await the next opportunity to try again. This is insanity. When one does the same behavior over and over expecting a different outcome one has stepped into the realm of addictive insanity.

I consider this phase of addiction to be one of the most tragic of them all. The addict comes to, what many in recovery call, the "jumping off place"—where using doesn't work anymore and neither can the individual imagine their life with or without the chemical. This is the pinnacle of misery, the crescendo of emotional desolation. This is full-blown addiction.

Phase Five: Imprisoned

Finally, all addicts eventually progress to this phase: imprisoned. Now they are addicted. The chemical they first fell in love with has left them. Their once found happiness has brought them to devastating new lows. The struggle, however, continues. When one is imprisoned by addiction, it has long ceased to be something they decided to do. Now it has taken on new meaning. It is something we must do, which is to say, no longer is it a choice, but rather a necessity (from the addicts perspective). Another way to look at this is as the phase of addictive maintenance. By maintenance, we mean that using chemicals is the norm, a norm which must be maintained, regardless of the cost. Hence, though the addict may no longer be receiving the perceived benefits of using, the habit must be perpetuated, if not for any other reason than it has penetrated the core of the addict's personality, in so far as, they identify themselves by their lifestyle in the same way an athlete finds self-definition in their sport or a business man in his job. Now the addict is subject to the addiction, imprisoned by the mad ruler ever more demanding and harsh. For the heroin addict, he or she is held hostage by the terrorist of intense physical withdrawal; therefore, for this person using is tantamount to merely feeling normal.

The more the addicted person struggles, the tighter the trap becomes. Like the "Chinese finger prison" otherwise known as Chinese handcuffs, when the fingers pull and fight, its grip becomes ever tighter. With each movement, the addiction is allowed that much opportunity to tighten its grasp around them. This phase is the ugliest of all. Here the addiction is king. Whatever the "master" desires, the addict will do. No matter who it will hurt or why, regardless of risk or consequence, the addict is now imprisoned to serve the chemical addiction. If it requires deserting responsibilities, jobs, and even family it must be done, the addict reasons. This phase is the culmination of the process, though an addict may, initiate the process again with different substances, this typically outlines the progress of addiction, at least in general terms. Please note these distinctions are not hard and fast categories that prescribe in absolute terms the way all people develop addiction, rather the above "phases" are offered in order to assist you in understanding the general contours of this perplexing disease.

Conclusion

The progression of addiction is catastrophic and heartbreaking. Nothing could be harder to watch. Nevertheless, each person who becomes an addict, progresses through these phases, or phases like these, into full-blown addiction. Each addict is a unique individual with specific circumstances, but addiction, in some sense, is static. It ever seduces more into its den to consume them for everything they have, much like a leopard who waits for her prey to move away from the group only to pounce upon its vulnerability.

Therefore, from our survey thus far, a few salient points may be asserted. Addiction develops progressively. During its course the person involved will become infatuated with the chemical(s). Then the potential addict will rendezvous with his "starry-eyed" lover to indulge in its hidden pleasures—only to later find that his precious lover has betrayed his trust through "infidelity." The following era of distress can be seen in his desperate attempt to recapture "the good 'ol days." Finally, these phases culminate leaving him utterly imprisoned to serve the chemical. He is trapped in a prison he unwittingly built himself.

Understanding the Addictive Personality

ADDICTION IS sustained by a belief system. In this section, we will explore the key beliefs of the addictive personality. These concepts form the cognitive structure that sustains addiction. These core values are generally characteristic in each addicted personality. Our understanding of these core beliefs will help us to understand more clearly the addictive personality.

Four Principle Warning Signs of Addiction

There are "warning lights" on the dashboard of your vehicle that will signal to those in the vehicle that there are internal problems. Indeed, just as your car has a "check engine" light, so also do your family members have "warning lights." These signs, for those who are attentive, signal you of internal problems before a breakdown takes place. In the case of automobiles they may enable you to avoid serious engine damage costing thousands of dollars. The same is true, yet infinitely more valuable, in the case of having an addict in the family. If you perceive these warning signs early enough and choose to address them, rather than dismissing them, you have the potential to save your loved one from jail sentences, institutionalization, and possibly even death; what is more, not only can you potentially save them from themselves, but one must also consider the incalculable savings of family anguish and financial hardship resulting from having an addict in the family. Undoubtedly, familiarity with these signs equips you to be pro-active rather than merely responsive to addiction.

Obsession—The first warning light of an ensuing addiction is obsession. Most forms of obsession are unhealthy, or at least if unchecked can be unhealthy. Obsession involves a constant thought or series of thoughts being replayed over and over. If your loved one is fixated on marijuana, those who use it, those who are trying to legalize it, the music that promotes its use, etc., that is obsession. Anytime we are consumed with thoughts of only one thing, it is obsession. One who is obsessing will arrange their schedule in order to accommodate the activity. In this case we're talking about using alcohol and other chemicals. When someone expressly schedules time or changes their entire life to accommodate a behavior, there is a high probability that it is problematic. On the other hand, persons, such as myself, in recovery have learned to "harness" my obsessions in healthy ways. So obsession by itself is only potentially detrimental, if directed towards negative behaviors and thought patterns. Thus, as you consider these "signs" remember that each one must be considered in light of the entire context of your loved one's life, personality, and behavior.

Negative Consequences—It should always be highly disturbing when a person begins to experience negative consequences from use. This, of course, must be clarified. For instance, there are degrees of consequence. In the case of a potential alcoholic, has he or she begun to experience consequences ranging in severity from hateful speech to those they love (i.e., saying things while drunk the person is regretful for later), punching holes in the walls of their room or home, threatening people, raging emotional outbursts, having accidents whether falling down or automobile related while under the influence? Also, negative consequences do not have to be legal. A common negative consequence for alcohol abusers is that they may be so intoxicated that they urinate in their bed while sleeping. Other negative consequences could be that a drinker always gets in brawls at the local tavern, or beats his wife, or sleeps around. These consequences can be observed in virtually every sphere of the person's life. Indeed, the list could go on infinitely.

The point is that someone who begins having these type consequences related to their use of chemicals should *evoke serious concern*. These are not acceptable behaviors and commonly both family and loved ones of addicts tend to make excuses for these consequences, blaming them on various factors, but all the while justifying the inappropriate behavior of the addict. Furthermore, if the potential addict gets arrested or faces suspension at work or school related to chemical use, this should be perceived with the same alarm a tornado or hurricane siren would arouse. Thus, be aware of your loved one's adverse consequences from using chemicals. This could appear in any of their personal relationships, whether with mother, sister, or girlfriend/boyfriend.

Another area that is commonly affected by using chemicals is vocational. Addictive persons' work performance will generally drop off significantly as the addiction progresses. Employers and co-workers are very aware of growing emotional disturbances and behaviors that people exhibit in the work place. However, sometimes, at least initially, the addict may experience potential success at work—indeed, if this happens they will usually correlate that with their use, thus perpetuating their own justification for using the chemical. Unfortunately, as one's addiction progresses, this success will diminish if not completely reverse. Also, money-management is a frequently mismanaged area in addicts' lives. During the progression of addiction, the addicted person could have significant negative consequences in their endeavor to manage their finances. Some even stop paying their bills and let them go delinquent. Others begin to liquidate their assets. What is important for you to understand is that addiction affects the pocket book of the addict. Be aware of negative financial consequences.

Mental health can significantly decline causing various disastrous outcomes. Usually this will manifest itself in depression, anxiety, fits of rage, etc. Sudden shifts in the emotional balance of your loved one should be a cardinal sign of trouble. While the problem may or may not be addiction, it is vital to be aware of. Drastic behavior changes and poor judgments are commonly associated with addiction. In the throws of an active addiction, the individual tends to make rash decisions without thinking through all the consequences. This is something to be on the look out for. If your loved one has been making many more poor decisions than what is "normal," there is cause for alarm.

Concluding our list of areas that might show forth negative consequences in the life of a possibly addictive personality is their physical health. Sometimes using different drugs can cause drastic changes in body weight. Other drugs that cause sleep deprivation may cause, what looks like dark rings under your loved one's eyes. Their face could appear "sunken in," as if they are sick. This is typical of certain addictions. You should always be aware of the physical health of your loved one if you are concerned they might be developing addiction.

Lack of Control—The development of addiction is most readily noticed by the expression of loss of control. For instance, if the family goes out to dinner and your loved one orders alcoholic beverages and seems to be unable to stop before becoming wildly intoxicated, that is evidence of a loss of control. This, at times, is one of the more difficult behaviors to recognize. This is not because the behavior isn't evident, but rather people have a tendency to downplay this type of drinking in general and thereby find it equally as easy to dismiss the behavior when people they love express it.

On the other hand, to some this is the attribute that most people judge addiction and alcoholism by. We find that to be inappropriate.

While lack of control is cardinal to addiction it is *not* the only indicator. If you notice your loved one using any chemical or exhibiting any behavior that they seemingly have no control over—you need to be concerned and address it. This can be food, drugs, sex, and anything else that in excess can be detrimental.

Denial—In this work we have dedicated a chapter to denial so here our presentation will be brief. Within the addictive context, denial is the inability or refusal of one to perceive the reality of their circumstances. Let's say for a moment your loved one obviously has a problem controlling their drinking or other behavior and you confront them. If they react as if there is *no problem* when there is enough evidence that clearly shows a problem does in fact exist, your loved one is probably in *denial*. For more information see chapter seven below.

Further Identifying Mentalities Associated With Addiction

Below we will interact with what I contend are identifying mentalities associated with addiction. By "mentality" I am referring to the general orientation, including both cognitive and behavioral, that an individual expresses towards the people around him or her. You will find these mentalities have been illustrated below by a general premise. This premise is meant to summarize the behavior/mentality pattern that is characteristic and may be used to identify the development or existence of addiction. Keeping with the general tenor of this work, we are seeking practical clarity, at the expense of "clinical" precision. These beliefs may vary in assortment per the individual. What will become obvious is the parallelism that exists between early childhood cognitive development and the addicted mentality, especially in regard to the latter's immaturity or failure to have progressed through the characteristic development of the former.

I Should Get What I Want All the Time

This underlying belief is the crux of addiction. Indeed, the deluded concept "I should get what I want all the time," stems from an underdeveloped maturity. It is at root fundamentally self-seeking coupled with the inability to perceive the feelings and needs of others. Thus, this type of mentality is inherently selfish. If you notice the person you love expressing "temper tantrums" such that a two or three year-old child might express, then you have encountered this identifying mentality. Undoubtedly, all people act selfishly and immature at times. However, a pattern of that behavior should be noticed as problematic. Developmentally speaking, this arises as the child is challenged by a world largely out of his or her control. Hence, they issue "demands" and seek to *control* their environment, which often proves to be quite a disappointing enterprise. This is further intensified with the new reality that life, as it were, seems not to "revolve" any longer around the axis of the child. Addicts tend to manifest this same attitude of preoccupation with having their desires and needs met prior to and often at the expense of others.

During the rearing of a two-year-old, it is the parents' responsibility to guide the child through this developmental stage. For the child to progress, he or she must embrace the reality that we don't always get what we want, exactly when we want it. The addictive personality though, believes that they *should* get whatever it is they desire in every given circumstance. Usually (though not always) the addicted personality will develop this core belief young and it will continue to grow as they become older. More often than not, it stems from a childhood without bounds. Loving parents generally attempt to give their precious child whatever he or she desires. Sometimes this can get out of hand. When it does, the child develops the concept that "I should get what I want all the time." This becomes a belief out of which they orient themselves to life.

Note also some of the consequences of thinking in this manner. If someone believes that their every want should be granted at all times, it leaves the door wide open to disappointment and resentment. If the this person believes sincerely that it is their "right" to get what they want when they want it, then in the case when their wants are not granted instantaneously, they feel cheated as if some great injustice has been done to them. Then (in the case of addiction) later in life they become raging tyrants when life doesn't go their way. These people inherently believe that what they want is of chief importance in the ranking of serious matters to be attended to. When their needs are not addressed immediately they become angry and sometimes violent. Others who don't act out become bitter and resentful. They quietly recede into their feeling of overwhelming injustice, as they tally the marks against those who didn't give them what they want when they wanted it.

Life Should Not Be Painful and Require Little Effort

The idea that "life should not be painful and require little effort" is the cornerstone of the modern American mentality. As a society, we seek out the easier softer way. We typically search for ease and shun pain. That which is painful is often considered "bad." The addicted personality functions on this premise. Addiction is a behavior pattern. Those who become addicted join themselves to an activity that is pleasurable. The next development, following that line of reasoning would be to resolve that anything outside the realm of pleasurable activity is un-pleasurable, and therefore, unacceptable.

Addiction is driven by desire for pleasure. To further explain this, a look at a concrete example will help. Let us consider the life of a cocaine addict. In the beginning, cocaine is the source of immense pleasure. Since life with cocaine is pleasurable, eventually one would come to reason that life without cocaine is void of that pleasure. This is then rationalized and justified internally by the addict, on the basis that they believe life should not be painful. Also, the addicted personality tends to embrace the thought that life should require little effort. Of course, this stands as the antithesis of the old ideal that "hard work pays off." It is typical for the addictive personality to be lethargic. More often than not, they expect success in life to fall in their lap. Thus, the addicted person's vision becomes deluded by flashy societal images of wealth and success being illustrated chiefly by a life of ease. A person who believes life should be relatively painless and require little effort, in my estimation, has an immature view of life. This mentality, alone, tells little about addiction, rather its benefit of signaling addiction will best be noticed as one attitude along with others described here.

I Am Not Good Enough

The belief that "I am not good enough" is a statement of insecurity. It evidences a poor self image. Nevertheless, addicted personalities frequently conclude that they inherently are not "good" enough to succeed at tasks or vocations such as school, work, or family, though the list could go on indefinitely. The problem in even discussing this matter is the arbitrary standard, often one derived from within the addict's own mind, namely, of *what* the standard of "good" or "enough" is. By convincing themselves of their own inferiority (or feeling of being "incomplete"), they set out to fail. Clinically, this would be one characteristic of "co-dependency." When one believes that within themselves they are incomplete, then it follows that they must "find" whatever will "complete" them. Thus, they embark upon a desperate journey to find the "missing" pieces.

Much of modern advertising supplements this thinking by promoting so many products to improve and "complete" individual's physical, emotional, and spiritual deficiencies. Indeed, the fundamental presupposition in most marketing is that without said product you are incomplete, therefore, you need product X. This is uniquely more intense in the addictive personality. It is not abnormal for the addict to be consumed with self-doubt and vulnerability. However, the manifestation of this typically perpetuates poor behavior and decision-making.

I Lack Something that is Available Externally

This rudimentary belief feeds addiction. The person who believes this is convinced that whatever is lacking can be found externally. The relation and overlap of this aspect to the former should be clear. This is expressed in sexual promiscuity, alcoholism, drug addiction, workaholism, etc. The sexually promiscuous person is found seeking "completion" or that "missing" piece in sex. Notice, the alcoholic, on the other hand, seeks to find what he is missing in the bottle. This belief fuels every late-night supplement commercial. "Product X in just one pill a day can improve your memory." "Lose weight while you sleep!" These are all ads that promote the idea of a "pill" (which, of course, is external) that will complete what is lacking. Addicted personalities are convinced that what they are "lacking" can be obtained externally (outside of themselves).

Whenever a person derives their source of pleasure outside of themselves, that individual has the potential to develop addiction. When someone is "incomplete" in their own person they are constantly dependent on outside things to have peace, joy, and happiness. In reality, my experience leads me to contend that happiness is a choice. Anyone who depends on other people or other things for their happiness is setting themselves up for disappointment. People are fallible and things don't always work out the way they are supposed to. So if one's emotional stability or "peace" is predicated upon variables that potentially could disappoint, balance is almost assuredly improbable. Thus, if you notice the one you care for to be dependent upon external things for fulfillment and joy, this should concern you. The more prevalent the pattern, the more cause for alarm there should be.

In brief survey of the above material, it should be clear the overlap involved in the areas of concern these premises illustrate. Therefore, to summarize if you notice your loved one operating with the mentality that they should always get what they want, that should be a sign of, at least, immaturity. Moreover, if that is coupled with the belief that life should be pain-free, they express a poor self-image, and are evidencing behavior which attempts to suppliment inadequacy externally, not only do you have a very unhappy person—you might be dealing with an addict. These souls feel mistreated, abused, and dejected. Even though they are unable to see the bigger picture, they still *feel* this way, and when dealing with addiction *feeling* takes priority of *reality*, in the mind of the addict.

Feelings are Bad

This belief is one that says effectively, "I should not feel what I feel." Usually this is sustained by the idea that life should not be painful. Feelings that are not pleasurable are dismissed as "bad." This trait empowers the addict to justify using external materials (i.e., chemicals, *et al.*) to suppress uncomfortable feelings. Often, the desire to "deal" with these feelings may be entirely natural, especially if they arise out of trauma such as sexual abuse, death, or other devastating circumstance. In fact, dealing with these feelings *is justified*, our concern is the *means* used to work through these feelings, which in the case of the addict is inappropriate. On the other hand, these feelings can merely be *felt or perceived*, which means: the individual may perceive certain events as "traumatic" emotional experiences; keep in mind, however, that other people may or may not consider these same events to be categorically "traumatic," which misses the point, from the addicts perspective. The issue is whether *they perceive* such events to be "traumatic" and thus evoke the desire to take steps in order that they might not have to experience the feelings.

The effect this has on the addicted person's behavior is that they, in turn, develop the pattern of suppressing their emotions. This might be expressed though the common conception of someone "drinking away" their sorrows or inhibitions. The local bars in your town are full of behavior like this. For instance, hypothetically, "Suzy" is a shy and attractive single woman. Suzy drinks in order to suppress her shy personality and become the outgoing life of the party. Running from one's own feelings is highly characteristic of the addictive personality. Since Suzy views her feelings as bad or something preventing her from a quality she desires, rather than working through her feelings, she merely sedates them. There are multitudes of ways this core belief can be expressed. Hypothetical Suzy is just one example of many. Feelings are generated by the human psyche and emotional network. Though there is great debate within the psychiatric community concerning methodology of counsel one should give concerning feelings, the simple premise we take here is that feelings should be considered neither qualitatively "good" nor "bad." This simply neutralizes the field so that people are permitted to feel, freely. This category, in so far as it signals an addictive mentality, is not always obvious, nor is it always indicative of addiction; therefore, exercise caution before to quickly assuming someone has this mentality, since it stands somewhat "below the surface" of a person's behavior.

Self-Obsession

Self-obsession is typical for the addictive personality. The addict most often is utterly consumed with thoughts about him or herself. Everything (from their perspective) has to be about them. They are constantly asking and wondering, "How does this benefit me?" However, the downside to this mentality is that it leaves little room within one's attention span for others. Self-obsession is what I refer to as the "me, myself, and I" syndrome. It is one of the most common traits of the addictive personality. When an individual is obsessed with self, their attention tends to be explicitly focused on those things that are pleasurable to self. Surely you can see how destructive this trait has the potential to be. Not to mention how unpleasant a person this would create. The self-obsessed personality typically is oblivious to the needs and concerns of others. This belief manifests itself in the line at the grocery store, in traffic, and numerous other places. People who hold to this view tend to be "accumulators." They are constantly gathering things and find momentary fulfillment in the acquisition of possessions, wealth, and self-gratification. For more on this mentality see chapter ten below.

Sense of Impending Guilt

This and subsequent categories will now begin to reflect less of a mentality and more of a characteristic emotive pattern, which may or may not be easily detected by others, especially by those without frequent exposure to the addicted person. The addictive personality many times will manifest itself in extreme defensiveness. The rationale underlying this is predicated upon an extreme sense of impending guilt. Characteristically, addicted persons many times will seem guilt-ridden. When they hear of someone being stolen from, they immediately feel guilty. When they hear of some other injustice they also feel guilty. This thought process is truly a tragic prison addicts generally keep themselves in. Since they knowingly persist in behavior that is inappropriate, most of the time against their own sense of morality, regardless of how skewed that may be, they usually feel guilty all the time. Their own addiction causes them to constantly violate their own conscience in order to appease the craving. As a result, the addicted person (generally) will at all times feel guilty or guilt ridden.

Difficulty Managing Anger

Addicted personalities usually have a great deal of difficulty in managing anger. Each addicted person constantly struggles with the great inner conflict: of doing what is known to be wrong in order to sustain what feels so right. They are also suffering the effects of consuming chemicals (i.e., drugs, alcohol, etc.). The chemicals themselves tend to generate their own levels of emotional disruption. The evidence of this is seen in explosions or episodes of anger. Anger, as here described, is the outward expression of inward turmoil. *Always, when confronted with someone who has rage/anger problems ask yourself—what feeling is this anger taking the place of?* In working with hundreds of families, whether adult or adolescent, I have always found that underneath anger problems lay intense feelings of hurt, insecurity, and other like emotions. Moreover, as addiction progresses, the addict will project a great deal of blame on others. This is an attempt to shift the blame to someone else. Once they shift the blame to others, they generally express this blame in anger. Therefore, pay close attention if your loved one expresses anger problems, it is certainly symptomatic of a problem, which might be addiction.

Depression

It is not surprising to find depression and the addicted personality operating simultaneously. Depression is a trait of the addictive personality. Of course, depression by itself is a mental health issue that could or could not have anything to do with addiction. Yet, rarely do you find the addictive personality without at least minimal depression. If depression did not exist before the addiction, it will be a result. The very chemicals themselves (alcohol, drugs, etc.) each cause unique side effects. Most of these include post-use depression. Chemicals that alter the way people feel also alter the chemicals in the brain, which control the human mood. When the neuro-receptors in the human brain function erratically, it causes a substantial chemical change in the brain that directly shapes human emotional and mental states of being.

Depression is not solely a characteristic of addiction, but it is a major indicator. In cases where it may be more difficult to determine whether a person is using drugs, it will be easier to notice the change in behavior.

Depression is one of the more "visible" types of psychological symptoms, since it affects a person's countenance and attitude.

Inner Tension

The addicted personality often wrestles internally with itself, causing inner tension. As stated previously, there is a major conflict between doing what the addict knows to be wrong and that behavioral necessity to satisfy desires that seem so "right." Inner tension usually consists of an inability to successfully manage emotions. The addicted personality has difficulty managing emotions effectively. This can be caused from excessive anxiety. Since addiction is partly psychological, that leaves much room for deficient systems of thought. Addicted persons often don't allow themselves the ability to *feel* their feelings, which has been touched on more extensively above. Therefore, this is probably a minor factor in regard to those which precede and follow it, nevertheless, it is one of many things that should one should be on guard for.

Dependency Needs

It is not abnormal for addicted personalities to be excessively needy, in terms of emotion. This means that it is not unusual for them to thrive on others' opinions of themselves or others' emotions toward them. Underneath all of this is insecurity that relates back to the belief discussed above: "I am not good enough." The addicted person may constantly be worried about what others are thinking or feeling. Usually, individuals who have dependency needs will be found asking repetitively; "Is everything okay?" and "You're not mad are you?" or "Did I do something to upset you?" This constant insecurity results from the dependence on others' emotions for them to feel "okay."

In early recovery this trait comes gleaming to the center stage. When an addict's chemicals are removed from the picture, the addictive personality turns to others to feel better. They attempt to please others and are concerned excessively with how others are feeling. They suddenly have the desire to become philanthropists with great burdens for those less fortunate. However, this is a guise in order to cover the deeper problem related to themselves.

Problems with Authority

The addicted personality, typically, will struggle, often greatly, with authority. To the addict authority represents control, which, for the addict, is *not* pleasurable. Their present addiction is sustained by over-indulgence in the given behavior. The presence of authority denotes accountability. Accountability, in turn, demands self-control. Self-control brings to the fore the possibility of less indulgence in the given pleasure. Therefore, authority stands in direct opposition to self-obsession, immediate gratification, and other traits of the addictive personality. The authority figure generally produces fear in the addicted personality because authority symbolizes those character traits which the addicted personality does not possess. To combat their own insecurity they become defiant to authority. Indeed, in the midst of this conflict other factors may come into play also, such as, the authoritarian figure becoming the proverbial whipping boy at which the addict may turn their blame, in order to, shift attention away from their own behavior. For more see "blaming others" below.

Deficient Coping Skills

Coping skills are an individual's emotional and intellectual ability to actively deal with adverse problems. The addicted personality has a deficiency or immaturity, if you will, in coping skills. They have trouble coping with everyday life. The problems that occur in daily life for any individual often produce great problems for the addicted personality. Dealing with loss, disappointment, and frustration become roadblocks that impede progress along the road of life. The addicted personality will have great trouble in coping day to day. They are deficient in coping skills.

Blaming Others

Addicted persons are professionals at blaming others. They have the unique ability to spot others' shortcomings and focus on them. This, usually, is to divert attention away from themselves, a theme which the reader undoubtedly is noticing as recurring with the addictive personality. Blaming others is both defensive and offensive in nature. It is defensive in the sense that it deflects or diverts attention. It is offensive, however, in that it is an attack against another person's character and ability. Usually this is a wedge that addicted persons drive between themselves and their families. The further the gap from family and self, the less authority and accountability the addict must deal with.

Since addictive personalities are guilt-ridden, they tend to blame others. This is done in an effort to feel better. It brings an inkling of relief to blame someone else. The heavy load of guilt for a moment lets up its incessant task. This trait seeks to emotionally wound as many people as possible for the aggressor is greatly troubled. It really comes from the childish theory, "If I can't have it, I'll make sure you can't either."

Immediate Gratification

Immediate gratification is what I like to refer to as the "microwave" syndrome. The reason I think of it this way is predicated upon the function of a microwave oven, which enables people to have push-button, instant solutions. The microwave epitomizes the quick-fix mentality. Addicted personalities are bound to instant gratification, which says, "Feel good *now*, and pay the price later." It's another fundamental of the addictive process. Heroin addicts use *now* in order to feel good immediately, not thinking of the long-term effects, namely, that using today will cause immense physical pain in withdrawal tomorrow. A credit card works the same way—charge now, pay later.

This is how addicted personalities function from day to day. They think: pleasure *now*, pay *later*. Oftentimes, however, we overestimate our ability to pay later. This causes us to mount an enormous debt in the long run from immediate pleasure in the present. It is this personality trait that makes addicted persons so prone to relapse. They don't think or take seriously the eventual consequences in relation to the present pleasure. Therefore, this could, from a different angle be a deficiency in appreciating behavior-consequence relationships.

Lack of Boundaries

Often the addicted personality will have trouble delineating where their own person ends and where others' begin. They lack proper healthy boundaries, in regards to interpersonal relationships. The addict isn't able to distinguish between his or her own person from others. At bottom, this is a dependency, or rather *co*-dependency issue. Persons who lack boundaries often say things that are socially inappropriate, especially in public situations. It may be common for the addicted personality to say things to others about personal issues in a way that crosses that person's "boundaries." What we mean is that at certain times and in specific contexts there are some subject matters that are inappropriate in conversation. This trait belies the addict's deficiency in knowing and handling mature social discourse and thereby having a common perception of what is right or proper to say, again highlighting their own lack of taking seriously others' boundaries.

Because of a lack of boundaries, it is not uncommon for the addicted person to have unhealthy relationships with loved ones. They will not have concrete individuality. The different personalities within their social sphere will "mesh" with their own, leaving them unable to appreciate proper boundaries in given situations.

Conclusion

All of these mentality/traits are characteristic of the addictive personality. They should guide you in discerning the different evidences of the addictive phenomena within the persons that you hold dear. Understanding is the key of greatest importance that will enable you to fight this battle. You must know that your enemy is addiction not addicts and thereby understand the disease's devices. Never forget, even though most of these beliefs are negative, that addicted persons are generally popular and even possess "magnetic" personalities, especially in social contexts. They are very pleasant to be around when not under the influence. They have great skills and abilities. Generally, most would assume these individuals are "good" people. Nevertheless, they have a bad problem. Now that you have an understanding of the addictive personality you are prepared to begin to—*Recover All!*

4

Toward a Biblical View of Addiction

FOR THE Christian, many dissonant voices clamor with "*the*" supposed insight into addiction, whether in relation to its cause, source, or underlying "power." Amidst these voices there are, *generally speaking*, two positions that attract the most attention, namely, the exclusively spiritual and the exclusively natural. Regarding the former, those who suppose that it is only a spiritual problem, attribute addiction to demonic or satanic powers. Indeed, in line with these contentions, this group formulates a solution, which is exclusively spiritual in nature. Juxtaposed to that position stands the opposite extreme, namely, that addiction is not a spiritual malady of any kind and merely relates to human psychology, behavior, environment, and nurturing. These latter fellows formulate a solution based exclusively in psychology, medicinal treatment, etc. Hence, these examples themselves yield an interesting fact—one's conception of the root issue of addiction, to a large degree, informs their practice in *treating addiction*. Where is the Christian left in all of this? Are those with the exclusively spiritual answer correct? Must the Christian eschew psychiatrists, therapy, and medicinal treatment (i.e., anti-depressants, etc.)?

These are issues that, as a Christian myself, I have wrestled with and I hope in what is below to offer a clear, biblically based median position. Essentially, as defined previously, addiction is *both* spiritual and physical—so, in a sense, we already have our conclusion. However, when we say "spiritual" does that necessarily imply that addiction is demonic, and if it is demonic, in what sense. For instance, does that mean some type of exorcism would suffice as opposed to therapy to remedy the situation? Though that may seem over the edge for most, there are good Christian people who have the conviction that addiction should be dealt with in that way.

In thinking through these issues, it might help to briefly articulate some of the problems of either extreme, that is, relegating addiction to either exclusively spiritual or natural arenas. The spiritual answer typically views addiction as *directly demonic* (i.e., incited by direct influence of a demon). The problem with this view is that it fails to explain and holistically address the genuine psychological, emotional, and environmental factors, which unaddressed deter the addict's chances of successfully abstaining from chemicals and recovering from addiction. That is to say, assuming direct demonic influence is true for the sake of argument, it is not at all clear that simply removing the demon would enable a person to work through their daily emotions and behavioral processes in a healthy way. Furthermore, believing this would seem to equip the addict with the ability to avoid taking responsibility for their addiction. Therefore, it is easy to see how this could be detrimental to the addict who is attempting to recover. Included in this category are those who suppose addiction is really just a "sin" problem, and thereby is demonic. We concur that in a secondary sense, sin is "satanically influenced" not to mention addiction frequently necessitates an individual's continuous "sinning;" nevertheless, sin itself remains a genuinely human malady imbedded within thought and behavior. So we fail to see how that gives any needed solution to the matter.

Conversely, to suppose that one can operate in a scientific world, as though a spiritual world does not exist, is to fundamentally *make a religious claim* and thereby take part in the religious project. All that is to say, neither option is valid—both regard two sides, of what we hold to be the same coin. Therefore, the popular idea that a neat separation of spiritual or religious concerns from scientific concerns is completely unfounded, not to mention unhelpful. In fact, that notion is gravely misleading. Spiritual matters, if they are genuine, which we affirm here are, happen to exist in dynamic unity with human thought and behavior and resultantly may not be separated, but rather should be addressed *together*.

With this in mind, we embark upon a journey together. In this chapter, we will deal directly with the issue of addiction from a biblical perspective and attempt to articulate, what I think the Christian Scriptures reveal concerning addiction, primarily focusing on the self-deception underlying addiction. It should be noted, contra much popular opinion, the Bible is *not* a textbook that speaks to every situation and circumstance. That is to say, the Bible does not *directly* deal with addiction. As the Holy Scriptures, Christian's (myself included) hold that the Bible communicates perfectly God's special revelation regarding himself, his historical interaction with his creation (i.e., humanity and the universe), and redemption from sin, by grace through faith in Jesus Christ.

Thus, there is no passage in the Bible that identifies or defines addiction. On the other hand, it could be argued that addiction *to sin* is one of the central themes of Scripture. However, for our purposes, below we will attempt to extrapolate some key ideas, which could help us understand addiction and the addictive process from a spiritual standpoint in light of the Bible's testimony. Therefore, what follows is entirely an *hypothesis* regarding how the Bible might inform one's understanding of addiction. Indeed, as the title to this chapter highlights, the information herein is offered in hopes that it will prove valuable as a beginning of sorts into further discussion and research regarding what the Scriptures have to say regarding addiction. The reader, then, must weigh the scriptural testimony and in so far as our conclusions adhere to it, agree or disagree.

It is my contention that much of what the Bible articulates concerning the thought or mental processes of spiritually darkened or lost persons, has direct relation and bearing upon the mental, emotional, and spiritual aspects of addiction, especially related to addictive self-deception. Thus, I will argue below that *sin* and *self-deception* have an intimate relationship. If one apprehends a better perspective of the self-deception of human sin, it will inform how we understand addiction. So using a construction motif—in the same manner that a building is constructed, we, too, will lay a foundation, raise a frame and, then put all the details in order to complete our work.

Pouring the Foundation

For a Christian to appreciate addiction, they must first understand more fully what the New Testament teaches regarding the great conflict between sinful humanity and her Holy God. Indeed, we must set forth some preliminary contentions or *presuppositions* from which the remainder of the argument will work. We affirm that the Scriptures teach that: 1) God created humanity in a *qualitatively good* moral and spiritual state, 2) humanity through breaking covenantal obedience to God incurred his covenant-wrath because of sinning (i.e., breaking covenant), 3) therefore humanity is incapable of fellowship with God on the basis of inherent depravity (namely, our sin *nature*), 4) Jesus Christ, the second person of the Trinity, took upon himself true humanity and bore the human penalty of sin in his own body upon the cross as part of the Triune God's eternal redemptive plan, 5) therefore, reconciliation with God and forgiveness of sin is available by grace through faith in the person of Christ to all humanity who will believe, 6) those persons who are unregenerate (or unsaved) may be said to be *lost* in regard to being reconciled with God. By unsaved we are referring to the estate of one who does not *salvifically know* Jesus

Christ. These presuppositions are, in my estimation, very fundamental evangelical Christian doctrines.

With the above presuppositions in mind, we must raise the questions: Why are the lost [persons] lost [spiritual state]? Or maybe to phrase it another way: what prevents the lost from seeing the truth? Why do unsaved people think the Gospel is foolishness? What is the real conflict?

To better answer these questions we must refer to the words of the Apostle Paul. In the second letter we have, which Paul wrote to the Corinthians, Paul addressed a concern of why spiritually dead people (namely, "lost") do not believe the good news of salvation in Jesus Christ. Paul states: "But even if our gospel is veiled, it is veiled only to those who are perishing, among whom the god of this age has blinded the minds of those who do not believe so they would not see the light of the glorious gospel of Christ, who is the image of God" (2 Cor 4:3–4 NET). What does Paul mean by "veiled?" Who is the god of this world? How does he blind their minds?

In this passage, "gospel" is used to describe the good news of the Kingdom of God and salvation through Christ. At its most simplistic conceptual level it contains the *basic facts* of the death, burial, resurrection, and ascension of Christ. We also note that Paul in Romans identified "the Gospel" as the power of God (Romans 1:16). So the truth about Jesus Christ is the power of God. The dilemma resides in the fact that it is *veiled* or *hidden to the lost*. The result of the "veiling" is that it (the Gospel) cannot be seen, which in this passage refers more to cognitive and spiritual "seeing" than to physical sight. Scripture, thus, describes a veil preventing the lost from cognitively perceiving the *light* of the Gospel. The veil obstructs the lost person's capacity to identify the truth of Christ.

The unbeliever is unable to understand the Gospel because the Light can't penetrate. Lenski's comments are helpful in this regard, "The mind is confronted with the divine reality, but instead of reacting as if it sees this reality, all its thinking and reasoning are as if it does not see at all."[1] So when unbelievers are approached with the Gospel of Christ, their mind and reasoning abilities act as if they haven't seen anything because of this veil. This appears to be good evidence that an aspect of the sinful condition is self-deception. That is to say, when one is involved in sin, in the case of this text—prior to being regenerate—they are unable, because of mental and spiritual self-deception to appreciate the truth of their condition and God's provision in Christ for them. As we continue, bear in mind that the importance is not in the state of being unregenerate, but rather

1. R. C. H. Lenski, *Corinthians,* 961.

the self-deception resultant from sin. Indeed, as we will see below, similar types of deception can and do manifest in the lives of believers.

Paul wrote in his earlier letter to the Corinthians, "But God chose what the world thinks foolish to shame the wise, and God chose what the world thinks weak to shame the strong" (1 Cor 1:27 NET). Even a cursory survey of most "special reports" on television concerning Christianity have a tendency to portray people of faith and sometimes even the convictions these people hold as foolish or ignorant. Therefore, many view Christianity as a crutch or ridiculous need of the individual to be "religious." In fact, that was my own perspective regarding Christianity prior to Jesus drastically changing my life and giving me the strength to stay sober. Actually, at least according to the Bible, unbelievers are (as I was) blinded from the truth because of the veil. Since the veil is preventing them from seeing the truth, it is foolishness or absurdity to them.

We find another example of this concept in Ephesians 4:17–18. Paul wrote, "So I say this, and insist in the Lord, that you no longer live as the Gentiles do, in the futility of their thinking. They are darkened in their understanding, being alienated from the life of God because of the ignorance that is in them due to the hardness of their hearts" (NET). Notice how Paul describes the difference between the saved and the lost. The lost have their understanding "darkened." Their minds are blinded from the gospel and their understanding is darkened. Indeed, Paul directly relates their spiritually darkened heart condition to their darkened understanding and vice versa. *Thus, for the Christian—psychology, emotionality, behavior, and religion are intimately connected, by design, and to treat one and not the others is problematic.*

Now in returning to our original text in 2 Corinthians 4:3–4: "[v 3] But even if our gospel is veiled, it is veiled only to those who are perishing, [v 4] among whom the god of this age has blinded the minds of those who do not believe so they would not see the light of the glorious gospel of Christ, who is the image of God" (NET). Who is the god of this world? What is the "mind," in this context? How are the minds blinded? The figure Paul is speaking about as "the god of this world" does not appear to be Jesus. He is referring, most likely, to Satan or more broadly to supreme evil power. Satan is the one who first tempted Adam and Eve in the garden. He is the father of sin and pseudo-"god" to those who are unsaved (see John 8:44). Paul here communicates that Satan *blinded* the minds of them who do not believe. It seems their own condition has inflated them as it were with self-conceit—or to put it in more familiar terms, the gospel is foolishness to them. Indeed, the sinful condition, namely, of self-conceit seems to itself be the "veil." If that, in fact, is the case it seems entirely possible that the root cause of the veil (self-conceit) preventing the lost from seeing the Gospel is most likely *pride*. Also, of grave significance is something provided in the broader context of this passage—that the solution to the veil is *divine action* [a sovereign work of grace] (v 6). Hence, the problem is not one that mere human ability on its own can remedy.

Along the same lines, Paul writes elsewhere to the Colossians warning his readers to be on guard for something conceptually parallel to that which we have just seen. In chapter two, starting with verse eight, he states, "Be careful not to allow anyone to captivate you through an empty, deceitful philosophy that is according to human traditions and the elemental spirits of the world, and not according to Christ (NET)." What is clear in this text is that Paul's concern was the leading astray of the Colossians by individuals who would brandish deceitful philosophies.[2]

He evidently supposes individuals *try* to *deceive Christians* with philosophies driven by *elemental spirits* or rudiments of the world. Let the reader key in on the phrase "elemental spirits of the world." This term is essential to our understanding of the text. The Greek term *stoicheion* (stoixei~on) refers to philosophic concepts and in some sense refers to transcendental powers active in the world.[3] Therefore, the ideas in view can have spiritual forces behind them. The word alternately can mean the basic components of something, which could equally be in view. In other words, it means the ABC's of something. These "ABC" principles form the fabric of a culture and dictate the thought patterns and resulting lifestyle of all members of that culture. Thus, *stoicheion*, in my estimation, constitutes the "god system" or "worldview" of a given culture. They form the basic strongholds that the Kingdom of God will challenge. The opposition

2. Parenthetically, I would like to clarify that some use this text against studying philosophy today. Though traditional philosophy at present is often hostile to religion that is hardly what Paul is speaking of here and therefore, is a terrible conclusion to draw from this passage! In fact, the New Testament would seem to argue that Christians should be deeply invested in understanding philosophy and being active in the academic community specifically as a witness for Christ. Paul himself quoted so-called secular philosophy of his day (see Acts 17:22–31, especially Paul's quotation of Aratus in v 28).

3. Though we have intentionally avoided extensive word studies here, this statement concerning stoixei~on is adapted directly from *the* authoritative lexicon in New Testament studies today: Walter Bauer, *A Greek-English Lexicon of the New Testament and Other Early Christian Literature*, rev. and ed. Frederick Danker, 3d ed. (Chicago: University of Chicago, 2000), 946. This term has been the subject of extensive debate through the centuries, for more information on the debate see Walter Wink, *Naming the Powers: The Language of Power in the New Testament, The Powers*, vol. 1 (Philadelphia: Fortress Press, 1984), 67–77 and Appendix 4.

does not specifically come from the individual, but from the "elementary principles." The veil that prevents the lost is rooted in pride and made up of a humanistic or a "man-centered" worldview.

In order to illustrate the importance of this, let's assume that there are only two worldviews.[4] On one hand, there is the biblical (God-centered) worldview, which stands mutually exclusive and diametrically opposed to the alternative humanistic (man-centered) worldview. By "centered" here we simply mean that in regard to thinking, either man or God is the final reference in predication (thought). Assuming that, we contend that what Paul is saying in 2 Corinthians about the lost being blinded in their minds is literally talking about their humanistic worldview preventing them from seeing the truth of the Gospel. The thought processes through which they interpret the world *are themselves the veil.* Or to say it another way, if man is ultimate in regard to authority and being the arbiter of reality and truth, then by default he is functioning as his own "god" determining right and wrong. This, of course, is quite reminiscent of the temptation in the Garden to be "as gods knowing right from wrong" (Gen 3:5).

The pride in humanity's heart prevents her from seeing the truth. Her own vain reasoning has philosophically explained away her account-ability to the Creator of the universe. Mankind, therefore, denies the truth for a lie (Romans 1:25). In sum, we have established that concerning the mental life of lost persons, according to the Scriptures, there is a self-deception, which cognitively functions against the individual's well be-ing—and ultimately eternal well being. As of yet we have not made the connection or relation of exactly how this condition of lost persons relates to addiction. To be clear, it is helpful to couch the subsequent discussion by clarifying what exactly we are *not implying.* Addicted persons are not necessarily unsaved. A person's salvific state in relation to Christ is not something directly related to addiction—which is to say, many Christian people become helplessly addicted to many substances.

Therefore, being a Christian of itself does not *solve* the addictive di-lemma. However, if the Bible does teach us about a cognitive self-decep-tion related to sin that directly interferes with an individual's ability to perceive reality truthfully, then we have a similar phenomenon to addic-tion (by analogy). Though the passages we have considered refer primar-ily to the lost, Paul was concerned that Christians in Colossae would be deceived by ideologies bound up with evil spiritual influence. I believe we can reason that, in so far as addiction has to do with indulgence in sin against God and our fellow humans, it is entirely possible that a relapse

4. "Worldview" will be explained further below.

of sorts into sinful self-deception might explain much spiritually about addiction. One thing is clear—the Bible seems very explicit in its regard for the importance of our thought life. Our ideas have far reaching consequences. Indeed, it aligns perfectly with Jesus' words, "Love the Lord your God with all your heart, with all your soul, and with *all your mind*" (Matt. 22:37 NET, emphasis mine). God doesn't just want your heart; he wants your thoughts, too. If we don't totally surrender everything, how can we ever be fully His?

Chiefly, we have asserted a few salient principles: 1) one aspectual effect of sin is that it blinds human thinking from God's truth, 2) sinful self-deception is seated in the mind (and in the case of lost persons—the spirit/soul), and 3) God is the only one who can pierce the veil. These building blocks are the foundation upon which we will raise the frame in our thought structure.

Raising the Frame

To frame a proper theory of addiction from a biblical perspective, we now can dissect the specific reasoning systems, which enable, foster, and promote addiction and addictive behavior. Hopefully, the previous section made clear some fundamental Scriptural truths in regard to the realm of thought. We have also established that *ideas have consequences.* Since ideas *do* have consequences, what are the ideas that foster addiction? Does the Bible talk about them? Though in an indirect manner, we think that it does.

As we revisit the elementary fabric of worldviews, they should catapult us towards greater understanding. A worldview in its simplest definition is conceptually (or properly *"noetically"*) *what is real.* It includes all the great ultimate realities of life pertaining to an individual's thought. The worldview each individual has shapes his or her beliefs. Beliefs happen to be the underlying system of values. In turn, human values are predicated upon what we believe to be good, beneficial, or best. Finally, human values determine our behavior. Therefore, behavior is the physical manifestation of an individual's worldview. (See diagram on next page.)

How we live, in actuality, is determined by our worldview. Assuming this to be true, you can certainly understand the serious implications of possessing a Christian worldview founded in the truth of the Word of God. It is also evident that the Lord and His Word are interested in what we think! This simple principle makes way for our next study. We will now explore some vital texts illuminating problematic systems of thought.

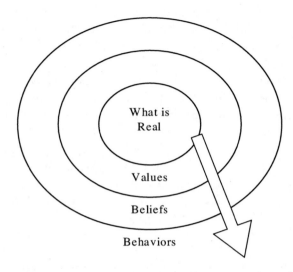

To further our insight of detrimental thought processes, we now will examine 2 Corinthians 10:3–5.[5] The Corinthians were notorious disputers amongst their own community. Paul was correcting them by pointing the finger at what appears to have been the root of the problem.

> For though we live as human beings, we do not wage war according to human standards, for the weapons of our warfare are not human weapons, but are made powerful by God for tearing down strongholds. We tear down arguments and every arrogant obstacle that is raised up against the knowledge of God, and we take every thought captive to make it obey Christ. (2 Cor 10:3–5 NET).

At the outset of this section, there will be a noted shift as we move forward from biblical texts pertaining to the lost. In this section, we will work with a text specifically written to Christians; therefore, the relation to addiction, while obviously not identical will be much easier to correlate. In the above passage, the believers in Corinth had allowed their focus to be swayed. Peripheral issues came to the forefront of dispute, blinding the believers to the real problem. The Corinthians had let personalities and other things gain importance while losing sight of the wickedness at work in the world often manifesting in people's behaviors, even within the Christian

5. Though this text is frequently employed in the teaching of "spiritual warfare," it is not our intention here to endorse "spiritual warfare" nor any of the theological aberrations and excesses that have risen out of that movement. We are merely concerned with what, if any value, this text might have to the present concern of addiction.

community. Paul says, in effect, even though we live in a physical body, our battle is not against physical enemies. For even though we are physical beings, our true battle is with those beings that *do not* have fleshly (physical) bodies. Since we are humans and live in human bodies it is easy for us to allow people and personalities to capture our attention and frustrate us. It is clear Scripture affirms that the real battle is not between people.

First our text made clear whom the battle involved. Now it explicitly defines our weapons while bringing our vision to a more precise focus on the source of our struggle. The weapons or battle equipment that we use are not carnal or human. What this means is that working out at the gym and having the physique of a warrior will not assist you in this regard. Physical muscles are of no benefit in this battle. The things that the "non-Christian world" considers vital to success in battle are without profit in this realm. Ironically, this seems somewhat counter-intuitive. We inherently associate physical strength with the ability to fight. Yet this text refutes our "traditional thinking" that our *might or power* is important, setting over against it the reality that God's power in our weakness—is true strength.

So we struggle against forces that are not human and as Christians have "weapons" that God has made powerful. The objective is the "tearing down" of strongholds. Metaphorically, the concept here is to impose a removal of evil influence from office or its *seat of authority*! We have capable power through God for the demolition of strongholds. God has made quite sure we understand that He has empowered us as New Testament believers with power to demolish and remove from power evil forces, in some sense. Also, please note that we are not here implying that the believer can wield his or her "faith" in some magical way to live victoriously, as is often espoused through the pseudo-Christian guise of faith-preachers on television. Rather, we are called to battle! Often this battle requires *suffering on the part of the believer for righteousness*. There is the guarantee of ultimate victory, in the end, whether or not that manifests in the present.

The issue then is the identification of strongholds. What are they? How do strongholds get established? We contend that a "stronghold" is conceptually a fortress or place of strength from which something or someone is controlled or held captive; indeed, it is a place from which one "holds" on to something. However, it seems to be metaphorical and in that sense probably refers to systems of thought, or possibly to worldviews. Let the reader recollect that in the context Paul is writing to Christians about their dealings with other Christians. *So obviously strongholds can influence*

45

or reside in believers! Parenthetically, let us note that we are not insinuating here any type of demonic possession.

Next, Paul argues, "*We tear down arguments and every arrogant obstacle that is raised up against the knowledge of God, and we take every thought captive to make it obey Christ.*" Here the Apostle articulates normative Christian praxis—the renewing of our minds and bringing our thought life in subjection to Jesus. In the midst of Paul's battle motif he makes an incredibly important point: our real spiritual battle is with anti-God thought and belief systems, that at times are even within believers.

This is stunning to think about. After a person has been saved, they have become a new creature in Christ. Old things have passed away and behold all things are new (2 Cor 5:17) . . . right? And yet, that doesn't address mental and emotional strongholds, which people bring with them. That is why every believer is called to "renew their mind" (Eph. 4:23) and "wash with the word" their thinking on a daily basis. Furthermore, notice that these things are *obstacles* to knowledge of God. We are battling exalted systems of thought, beliefs, and philosophies. It should be obvious how this correlates with addiction. Paul is here describing a battle with thoughts that are fundamentally at odds with truth or reality (i.e., the knowledge of God). These thought processes are in direct opposition to the truth, which makes them, reducing them to their lowest common denominator—lies.

Therefore, reviewing for a moment the territory we have covered thus far, we have established: The believer is in a "war" (figuratively). This fight has an enemy that is not other humans. The real enemy is in the minds of people, even believers. The real enemy is comprised of philosophies, beliefs, and thought systems that attempt to usurp God's Word. Believers must rely on God's power in action through his Spirit to destroy and remove from office these systems of thought and belief that oppose God and truth.

How do we do this? How do we enforce victory and successfully remove from office these wretched systems of belief? *We must bring these thoughts into captivity to obey Christ.* That is the means to recovery, both from the remnants of our previous sinful nature and also the remnants of *addiction.* One root *aspect* of sin, at least in this context, is wicked *belief structures within the mind.* The root of these structures is pride! These things oppose God. God demands their removal from office and submission to His lordship. Does He desire us to address just some strongholds, when we are "ready" to change? No. He demands the overthrow of *every* stronghold.

Finish Out

In every building project there is a "finish out." This is the phase of development when the structure finally journeys from type and foreshadow to take its finished form. Along our journey, some of you may be wondering how any of this biblical excursus has anything to do with addiction. It, in fact, has everything to do with addiction. The perplexing thing to most Christians is how "good," God-loving people become ensnared in the trap of addiction. Sure the answer is as simple as "sin," but that really doesn't comfort those who are earnestly asking the question, especially in a cultural climate that has largely abandoned the doctrine of sin to begin with. Chemically dependent people cross the threshold of "self-control" into dependence and addiction. So the whole idea that telling an addict to "just quit" using, or for that matter, just stop sinning, isn't as easy as it might sound.

When we approach the subject matter from a biblical perspective, we are able to see the source. Addiction is sustained by a series of "strongholds," if you will. These are literally fortresses of thought—systems that stand in opposition to God. They are elusive. The task of their overthrow is not so simple, neither is it the same as hunting a visible enemy. This enemy hides within the recesses of the human psyche. Since the adversaries have complex camouflage, it requires the power of God to flush them out and demolish them. It is necessary at this point to caution the reader. As mentioned in the beginning of this chapter, there are two extreme sides to this subject. We hope here to put forth a "balance" of the two. The reader must beware of spiritual extremists who demand that the *only* solution is spiritual.

We affirm that addiction is a spiritual problem. These strongholds (thought processes) are many times demonically based. That is not to say, that an addict has a "demon" as though some type of exorcism would heal the situation. Moreover, one would be *unwise* to limit themselves to spiritual remedies only—which in the final analysis, taking into account Scripture, fundamentally undermines the Christian approach, which *should be open to virtually any form of help in this matter*. Experience has proven in my life (and many others I've worked with) that the entire problem of addiction, while being a spiritually originated malady requires the rehabilitation of the "whole" man—spirit/soul (mind, will, and emotions) and the body. While it is unwise to jump to the spiritual extreme dismissing non-spiritual rehabilitation, it is also severely detrimental not to address the spiritual root of addiction. Obviously, God has a great deal to say about what we think. He requires believers to submit the entirety of themselves to Him.

We have gathered from our texts seven key elements that need to be retained in developing a balanced biblical perspective of addiction.

1. *Chemical use is the outward expression of an internal problem.* Sadly, so many well-meaning individuals think the bottom-line solution to cure addiction is *stop* using. While without question the fundamental principle of this thinking is correct, it stops *far* short of a real long-lasting solution. Addiction (in its most basic forms) is found disguised in distorted systems of thinking which stem from an inaccurate perception. The actual use of chemicals is a *symptom* of the problem. The problem is internal. More specifically, it's spiritual, mental, and emotional.

2. *Addiction as with any malady has a remedy, which God can provide through Scripture, Christian people, and not least of which would be His direct intervention.* God has supplied Christians with Scripture. The Bible may not always tell us what we want to know. It does, however, tell us everything we *need* to know for salvation and godly living. The Bible gives us the "roadmap to recovery." Never forget recovery is God's idea. Christianity is about recovery, in many senses of the word. Furthermore, Christian people can genuinely help in a variety of ways, not the least of which is prayer and support in your struggle. And without question, God can intervene supernaturally, *or* his supernatural deliverance could come through a treatment program, counselor, or even a book like this one, which God chooses to use for His purposes. So we contend you should be *open* to God's working through a variety of means.

3. *Deception blinds the minds of those who are perishing in it.* Once the addiction becomes a full-blown active process, it is sustained by deception. We must always realize that in the same way that the lost are "blind" or "veiled" to the gospel, addicts are "blind" to the reality of their problem. We should never point our "attack" toward a lost person, in some strange attempt to force them into the kingdom, and neither should we attack addicted persons. We are to direct our efforts to the "veil" or "blinder." Always remember the addicted are blind. This *does not* absolve them from responsibility. Yet they are unable to collectively reason rationally. You will find often that dealing with an addict is reminiscent in many ways of dealing with a developing child, usually around three years of age.

4. *Addiction is one of the many evils that spring out of strongholds in the human psyche.* Virtually all behavioral disorders find their roots in strongholds. Alcoholism and drug addiction are no different. While the source of addictive thoughts obviously are in the psyche, they are only one of many problems that could be stemming from these strongholds. One would be unwise to think that once the sustaining belief systems of addiction were addressed there might not be some other detrimental thought processes (i.e., pride, lust, greed, etc.).

5. *We are not "battling" against the addict or the drugs, but the strongholds, which foster the addiction.* This point cannot be emphasized enough. It is far too easy to point the finger at the addict rather than painstakingly root out the source of the problem. Our battle is with the vain philosophies that feed a person's continual chemical use. When attended to properly, the overall long-term possibilities of recovering are, in fact, encouraging. Parents and family members, your loved one has not become a "bad person." They simply have adopted or been taken captive by ungodly thinking. Simple discipline such as grounding, taking away privileges, etc. will not solve the problem. It has a deeper root. Together, the power of God through you, along with ministers, and trained professionals, *can* demolish these areas. The Word of God is and must be the source of both hope and victory to the Christian in all their affairs, including rehabilitation for addiction.

6. *Recovery is the product of taking captive every thought, philosophy, and belief system and bringing them in submission to the Lord Jesus, the author of all Truth.* Recovery is the lifestyle that is produced from strongholds being subdued. It commences when these belief systems are brought into submission to Christ (Remember, Jesus is truth and righteousness). When the righteous Jesus reigns over your thoughts, your actions can't help but follow. All behavior flows out of our thinking. "For as he thinks in his heart, so is he"(Prov. 23:7 NKJV). How we think determines what we say and the destiny we walk toward.

7. *Strongholds not addressed are like weeds; they will continue to spring back up until your root them out.* Anyone who assumes they have thoroughly dealt in any way with addiction, yet has not addressed the thought processes of the addict, is sorely mistaken. This person is on a collision course with the harsh reality that they must address the spiritual malady. Even though the A.A. (Alcoholics Anonymous)

program is given much bad press, (regrettably, in the church) it maintains in it's *The Big Book*® that alcoholism is a spiritual problem that requires spiritual treatment. Recovery requires spiritual deliverance, healing, and restoration. Without it, the "whole" of the problem has gone untreated.

5

What Are the Signs of Drug Use?

THE MOST frequently asked question and toughest to comprehensively answer that parents pose is, "How will I know if my child is using drugs and alcohol?" Few questions bring as sharp a knot to the stomach of most parents. Though it arises so frequently, it is fraught with difficulty due to the fact that there are so many variables. That is to say, addictive processes by their nature are often shrouded in secrecy, lies, and deception. That, coupled with the reality that a loved one may present themselves one way in a certain context while essentially living an alternative life before others, further contorts the situation. Indeed, for those who have no experience with addictive behaviors it is hard to imagine how such a person would ever recognize the warning signs, especially if *real* warning signs were somewhat more subtle than those presented on film or television. Furthermore, American society has grown ever more individualized creating a huge gap between parents and children. What is more, the rapid advancement of society both technologically and otherwise makes the task of keeping up with a young persons lifestyle and influence ever more difficult for adults. Only recently have people been realizing that parents have to be conscious of who their kids are talking to on the internet, cellular phone text messaging, and what music they are listening to on their IPod™.

Amidst these complex issues remains the reality that *every parent* must be conscious of the influences and behaviors of their children and family members. Indeed, they must always be prepared to ask themselves if their loved one might have an addictive problem. Addiction transcends race, color, creed, age, education, economic status, and anything else that separates one human from the next. Parents and family members are oftentimes the *last ones* to recognize it, even when it is obvious to everyone else. This touches on denial, a concept dealt with in a later chapter, but for now it is necessary to tell you that loved ones often see the signs described in this chapter and merely relegate them to other causes, simply because they don't want to or are unable to face the facts. Do not be one of the thousands of tragic stories; being proactive and overcautious far outweighs the alternative which might include the death of a person you dearly love. Like cancer, addiction progresses, and if untreated it is almost certainly terminal. This is a hard truth to come to grips with. What is even harder, though, is to stimulate people to actively stay conscious of its development.

In this chapter, I will attempt to assimilate the most accurate and important warning signs a parent should look for. Of course, a topic such as this could fill scores of volumes with countless pages. Despite the broad nature of the subject matter, we will attempt to cover the fundamentals. This should assist most people in determining whether or not their loved one is, or might be, using and/or abusing chemicals.

Taking Off the Blinders

For one to have an adequate understanding of drug use, one must first realize that drugs and alcohol are the expression or physical manifestation of a problem, a lifestyle, or an addiction. Many times these three elements mesh together so closely that it becomes difficult to differentiate between them. Drug and alcohol use have both a distinct culture and lifestyle. From this perspective there are many different "brands" of drug users. The last time you were in a convenience store, even if you were not a smoker, it would be hard for you not to be inundated with the immeasurable variety of cigarette brands. The drug culture and lifestyle is virtually the same. Addicts come in all shapes and sizes. Some have wild hair, a plethora of piercings, and an array of tattoos, whereas others are high-class business executives, educated at the finest schools. So to stereotype addicts by what they look like, where they live, or what kind of music they like, would be a *catastrophic mistake*. Before we can move into what to look for, we must look inward.

First, you must remove from your mind any stereotypes you may have about what "drug people" look like. This may seem elementary. Yet most people, whether conscious of it or not, have certain stereotypes. To be a well-informed and aware family member or friend, you must not be *deceived*. Deception starts with you. One central and common mistake people make is the perpetuation of the false idea that "a little pot smoking" for the experimental teen is not anything to be concerned about. The present situation regarding the potency of substances and the associated culture have far surpassed, in severity, anything previous generations experienced. The marijuana on the streets today is 400% more potent than the marijuana commonly confiscated in the 1960's. The cocaine and heroin in circulation today is so much more potent than the drugs used in past generations that it's staggering. Even "hip" parents who think they are in touch with their teen can be deceived! Deception is a major battle that is usually fought silently, but its implications are far-reaching and have the potential to devastate a family. You must be cautious not to become deceived.

To prevent from being deceived as parents and family, we must embrace three simple principles.

Principle One: Realize that your perception is fallible. Just because you don't visibly see smoke, does *not* mean there isn't a fire burning in the house. All humans perceive reality from an internal vantage point. Often we see and hear what we expect and want to, not necessarily what is real. Indeed, it is entirely possible for our minds to reinterpret simple data in a completely contrary-to-reality manner. Thus, two people might witness a car accident from two different sides of the street, each witnessing different aspects of the same event. Therefore, each witness might attribute the cause of an accident differently because of their vantage point and the way their minds process the data. This is a disadvantage which all humans take part in—namely, our own subjective perception. However, typically we come to rely on our perceptions, sometimes more so than we ought to. It is this problem which is being addressed here. You must recognize that regardless of your involvement in your loved ones life, it is *entirely possible* that you are not perceiving everything. Indeed, you might be getting the "wrong reading" completely. Therefore, an old adage is helpful in this regard: "Don't rest on your laurels." This is foundational and serves as the first vital concept in avoiding deception. In the same way that a pilot relies on his instruments, you, too, rely on your senses, but instruments (if not set properly), will *mislead* the pilot. Don't become oblivious to the possibility that there may be something going on that *you don't know about.*

As a minister, I was serving in a local church as a youth pastor. A young man in my youth group was a star high school football player. He had a brother one year older than him, who was in high school as well. Tragically, his mother found the older brother dead one afternoon in his room. He had begun experimenting with heroin. His death was a result of an overdose on heroin. This young man only experimented with the drug two or three times in his life, and then through an accidental overdose died. There were no warning signs, at least to his immediate family who lived in the same house. His mother wasn't even sure if he ever had tried drugs. She certainly had no reason to suspect that her child might be using drugs, much less hard drugs like heroin. As horrible as it sounds, this story is more commonplace than often goes reported in the local news. In fact, this prominent story got less attention than the nightly lottery numbers.

Don't think for a second this occurred in a poverty-stricken area. This happened in one of Dallas/Fort Worth's premiere suburbs. A place where families from all over desire to live because it is supposed to be "free" from this type of problem. To put the suburb in perspective, the lowest income housing in the entire city were apartments that cost more monthly than most upper-middle class mortgage payments. Therefore, *no neighborhood or social class is exempt.* The drug problem is real. In fact, often drug use is more prominent in middle to upper-middle class neighborhoods than in the "ghettos" where most people perceive the drug problem is. This mother will live the rest of her life in the absence of her son. She was a loving mom who cared deeply for her family. She didn't neglect her son by any means; she was simply caught off guard. One could even say that she was *deceived* by the assumption that everything was okay. She thought drugs weren't a problem in their neighborhood. She never would have imagined her son would use heroin. Don't let deception rob you of the ones you love. Realize that your perception is fallible, and always stay open-minded in regards to the possibility that this plague might find itself on your family's doorstep.

Principle two: Facts don't lie, people do. Be careful not to let the simplicity of the principle allude you to its importance. The harsh reality in life is that good people sometimes do bad things. People lie. Sometimes these people who lie happen to be your family. Virtually, all parents inherently trust their children. Common sense would seem to say, "I raised them, and I know they are generally always honest with me." This kind of thinking, of course, is quite compelling both intellectually and emotionally. That, however, is what makes this mentality so dangerous when addiction infiltrates your family.

Sometimes the hardest thing for a parent or loved one to do is face the facts. Addiction, as with any illness or spiritual malady, has symptoms. The identification of these symptoms is crucial to the successful treatment of the problem. For instance, women over a certain age are required by their doctor to have annual breast exams. If a woman who stayed alert to the symptoms were to find a lump in her breast months prior to her exam, it would greatly increase the odds of her cancer being successfully treated. Ironically, in that same situation it would be ludicrous for that same woman to pretend she didn't find the lump. That very idea simply sounds ridiculous, doesn't it? As silly as that example is, people do that very thing everyday. They put on blinders in regards to their child, spouse, or family member's addictive symptoms! Thus, people tend to relegate the facts to the periphery, explaining them away in order to believe their loved one. However, facts don't lie, people do.

It is also important to note that lying and addiction go hand-in-hand. The most honest people in the world, when they become addicted, become conniving, manipulative liars. This is not to say that an addict can never be believed, but an addict in active addiction will be notorious for lying. Often it takes time to notice the large web of deception which addicts create, at least in early addiction. When things continually seem contradictory, out of place, and you begin to perceive that you are being told lies you should be concerned. Deception is one of the greatest symptoms. Not only is the addict deceptive in their interactions with others, but they often are deceived themselves. Most addicts convince themselves that there is nothing wrong, even some of the most severe users. Thus, since a major factor of addiction is self-deceit, then logically, people who are deceived themselves will deceive others both consciously and unconsciously. Again, lying is a symptom of addiction, yet it needs to be reiterated that addicts who lie should not be thought of as "bad" people.

So in the case of chemical dependency, when you begin to notice various things not adding up with your loved one's stories concerning where, when, and why they do things, you should give priority to facts which can be grounded. Thus, the principle that "facts don't lie, but people do," simply means that you need to be on guard not to miss the facts for the lies or to put it another way, "don't miss the forest, for the trees." When it comes to addiction and those who are chemically dependant, their behavior should exemplify their intentions. Yet this is often not the case. Addicts tend to know all the "right" things to say, but day after day do the wrong thing. This highlights the disjunction between intentions and practice. Thus, as a loving and responsible person in the addict or possibly addicted person's life, you must be willing to face facts even if it means being confronted with the possibility that the person you care about has been lying to you. We must not let false assurances of honesty cause us to miss the harsh reality.

Principle three: Stay involved, stay alert. One of the most essential things any parent and family can do for a loved one is to stay *involved* in their lives and to stay alert to their disposition. Part of staying alert means knowing what to look for and staying current with the signs and symptoms of drug and alcohol abuse. Staying involved means asking questions. Questions can make the difference between detection and death. A family who doesn't ask questions is a family headed for deception. Somehow our culture today has placed an inappropriate premium on "privacy." This is not helpful at all to preventing a loved one from deceiving you.

It was commonplace that I would receive calls to the House of Isaiah men's recovery program admissions office, from mothers, sisters, and wives who knew in their heart that something was wrong. All the indicators were there, but the individual would evade facing the issues because they would skillfully defer questions. For a moment, let's think through some implications from this type of deception. Meet Carl, he is 28-year-old man that recently went through a rough divorce. Presently, he has moved home with his father and mother. He has been out of work for the last 4 months. The divorce was very ugly, pulling the kids in two directions. Carl has been so emotionally crushed he hasn't been able to hold down a job. He has recently started coming home at all hours of the night and sleeping all day. He says he's looking for a job. Yet each night he comes home with the stench of whiskey on his breath, intoxicated, and angry. Finally, Carl's mother demands that if he is to stay in her house, he cannot drink.

Now when Carl comes home, his mother asks him where he's been. Carl retorts, "out." (As if his mother couldn't have figured that much out!) When she questions him further, he reacts defensively to the extreme, wondering what gave her the right to "pry" into his personal business. Now this example could apply to man or woman, teen or adult. The key is Carl doesn't think his family has a "right" to ask him questions. However, the reality is that Carl lives under their roof, eats their food, and uses their money. The parents and family have *all the right* to ask any question they like. Carl has a mistaken concept of "personal rights."

The sad part of it is, many parents in this position back down to the addict. Addicts have a profound ability to twist the truth in order to manipulate their situation. The issue to Carl's mom was his whereabouts. The desire for knowing this information was not for any other reason than love and concern. Carl manipulated the situation by turning it into a "right of privacy issue" as if his mother had done him a great injustice. Carl redirected the entire event by calling into question his mother's motive and right to ask. Hence, by a sleight of hand, Carl shifted the attention from the real issue to something else.

Social Indicators

Drugs and alcohol have their own sub-culture with many different faces. We will now begin to look at some of the social indicators associated with drug and alcohol abuse. Let us make certain that we understand that some of the issues brought up in this section are *not* the sole determining factor of addiction or abuse, but can and do directly relate in some form or fashion. Many subjects and behaviors covered in this section are only secondarily indicators of abuse and addiction; that is to say, one single factor by itself doesn't always mean *addiction* or *abuse*. Therefore, let the reader exercise caution and wisdom before to hastily coming to the conclusion that a person is an addict or not. With that said, we will cover three major social areas, which will show us indicators of the drug culture, which in turn will point us in the direction of abuse. As the old saying goes, "If you hang out in a barbershop long enough, you're bound to get a haircut."

Addiction deals specifically with behavior. What an individual does with their time indicates their interest and priorities: *that which we love, we spend time with*. This fundamental principle is established in the mind of every child. The natural equation is: TIME=LOVE and LOVE=TIME. If you say you love me, but don't spend time with me, your words are empty and meaningless. Once we realize the practicality of this principle, we can understand the importance of with *whom* and *what* people do socially. The first social area we want to focus on is music. Music is one of the most influential medias available. For many, music is a refuge from the hustles and bustles of everyday life. For others, it is a great accompaniment to a workout or yard work. Virtually all people are directly affected by music in some way.

Since music is so prevalent in our culture and because music takes on so many faces, we will only be focusing on a few areas. Our concern is the lyrical content, motive, and predominate listening audience. There is nothing inherently wrong with virtually any type of music in any way. Lyrical content has been a very controversial issue on many occasions. So to be frank, we are not in any way attempting here to establish the "right" or "wrong" music. What we are going to do is look at a handful of genres and the specific messages they typically promote. There is little doubt that some of the generalizations made in this section will not be without disagreement. Therefore, the reader, again, is cautioned to use this information as a guide, not a *rule*.

The genres that endorse illicit drug use, sexual immorality, and crime characteristically go hand-in-hand with the activities they endorse. Meaning, if I am using marijuana, most likely I will choose a music type that encourages my lifestyle. If I listen to "gangster" music, then most likely I will walk, talk, dress, and act in a like manner. If I listen to "club" music, my lifestyle (more often than not) will also reflect the music I listen to. Or conversely, it is also possible that individuals, because of their lifestyle and behavior choices gravitate toward music that coincides with their behaviors.

So as family members we want to ask ourselves: "What music does my loved one listen to? What are the songs about? What do the songs promote?" We want to be alert to music that explicitly endorses illicit drugs. "Gangster rap" and hip-hop, though not exclusively by any means, are notorious for promoting drug use and drug dealing as a viable means of making a living. It should be a concern on any parent or family member's mind if their loved one is listening to *any* type of music promoting immoral and or illegal behavior.

A good example concerning musical motive of a genre is "techno/ trance" music. This genre is very different from rap and metal, and it serves as a media to another sect of the drug culture known as "ravers" or "party kids." A rave is an all-night party, commonly held "underground" on the weekends. They generally last all night long and thousands of young people attend to partake in the proverbial festival of chemicals with such drugs as: LSD (acid), ecstasy (designer drug), Ketamin, and a plethora of various other illicit drugs. The music itself has few if any lyrics. It usually is a blend of fast paced beats blended with electronically generated sounds from keyboards, records, drum machines, *et cetera*. This music actually can be quite entertaining, and again the *music* isn't the problem. We just want to be aware that characteristically those who listen to it, often are drawn to it by the lifestyle and party scene that it represents. Or in my case, I continue to listen to it in sobriety because it is upbeat and generally without lyrics, thus it can be listened to while doing other things. This highlights the point that merely listening to a type of music, *could*, but does not imply drug or alcohol use!

Finally, a family member needs to be aware of the predominate listening audience of a select type of music. Every genre has a select audience. For instance, techno music is associated with rave parties or the club scene. If a parent was oblivious to the fact that rave parties exist and are common in every major city in the United States, that same parent would miss the "indicator" that their child might be involved in rave parties and the drug use that goes on there. The music your loved one listens to is a voice into their lives, whether positive or negative. It has been my experience that whether people choose to admit it or not, what you listen to affects your thinking, emotions, and behavior—especially in regard to lyrical content.

Another significant social indicator parents and family must be aware of is manner of dress. Does your loved one dress cleanly and neatly? Or rather do they put little emphasis on personal hygiene and appearance?

These things alone do not indicate drug use, but they can go hand in hand. Does your loved one wear "gothic" style (all black, black makeup, chains, etc.)? This kind of dress generally reflects their emotions and characterizes some kind of emotional instability, it may not be addiction, but it definitely is something.

Along the lines of reinforcing our principle of "time equals love," what are your loved ones interests? What or whom do they spend time with? The answers to these questions will assist you greatly in being alert to the signs of developing addiction, depression, or other malady. We truly are our brother's keeper; we are responsible to notice the social indicators in order to help the people we know.

What Are You Doing?

Next, it is essential for our study that we address behavior, since addiction is primarily behavioral. Every parent wants to know what to look for. So far, we hopefully have provided you with a structural outline of key factors to look for. Here we will examine specific behaviors that are characteristic of chemical abuse and chemically dependent persons. Anger is certainly not exclusive to chemical dependency; however, most users exemplify anger. Some harbor past resentments. Others become very impatient and dissatisfied. Normally, people who choose to use chemicals to change the way they feel are running from something. So it is simply logical to them to be angry with the issues they are running from.

Chemical use has a unique ability to cause the individual to have little patience with themselves or others. Again, the actual use of chemicals is evidence of a deeper emotional dilemma. Those who use stimulants often experience a very rough emotional dive after use. Stimulants instantly make them feel euphoric and energized. Then the effect wears off and an abrupt emotional nose-dive occurs. Typically, chemical use will cause dramatic changes in attitudes and behaviors of individuals. If your loved one has had a pattern of "normal" behavior and suddenly there is a shift in behavior and attitude—that definitely warrants further investigation. Any dramatic sudden shift can be cause for alarm.

Isolation is another pattern that needs to be watched for. Sometimes a very flamboyant and alive teenager will suddenly become reclusive. This may not be a sign of drug use, but it definitely could be. Addiction is fostered in *distant* relationships. The further your loved one distances themselves from intimacy with you, the easier it becomes to facilitate chemical abuse. Have you ever noticed that, generally speaking, people who are doing something wrong are always defensive? They are. This is why, most of the time, chemical users become very defensive about their behavior and actions. They seem to find it necessary to always be on the defense since deep down they are aware that their behavior is unacceptable. None of these factors alone determine the use of drugs. However, these behaviors usually always accompany it.

Individual Drugs

In this section, we will look specifically at individual drugs, their aliases, specific items evident in their use, physical symptoms of being under the influence, and common behaviors attributed to use. By its nature the information is constantly influx—that is, terminology changes virtually everyday. Furthermore, some of the physical signs described below are not meant to supplant or correct any medical documentation, rather the information is meant to be a *guide* not an authoritative medical account of the problem. Thus, our concern here is practical. This section is a compilation of my own experience as an addict, my experience working in the field, and my own study of the subject matter distilled for simplicity.

Cocaine

Cocaine is a stimulant that directly affects the nervous system. It creates an instantaneous euphoric experience, which is very powerful, yet short-lasting. Cocaine affects the heart significantly in that it causes the heart to beat multiple times faster than normal increasing the risk of cardiac arrest. This drug is extremely addictive in nature and causes severe emotional and mental withdrawal. The physical withdrawals are few, which is to say, the body does not seem to go through noticeable withdrawal. Many adults who are not familiar with cocaine get confused when the term "crack" gets brought up. Cocaine is used in a variety of ways. However, for our study we will look at the three most prevalent methods of using cocaine. These three different ways depend upon the *form* that the substance cocaine is in. For instance, the first and most common way to use cocaine is by "sniffing" or "snorting" the cocaine powder.

The second most common way cocaine is used is by smoking it. This is usually called "free basing." If the powder cocaine is mixed with baking soda and water it can be hardened into a "rock-like" substance. This new substance is commonly called "crack cocaine." Crack is one smokable form of cocaine. This method simply allows the cocaine to enter the bloodstream via the lungs. This method has a more powerful effect because it reaches the brain faster—within seconds.

Thirdly, cocaine is injected. This is made possible due to its water solubility. (This also means it is not stored in fat cells, so within three days cocaine is undetectable in a urine drug test.) Since it so easily dissolves in water, this method is relatively simple in regard to the process of transferring it to water and then injecting it. This method simply mixes the cocaine substance in a small amount of water, and then is injected directly into the vein. Regarding effect, this is the most potent method of use. Since the cocaine is not filtered at all through the lungs or sinuses, this gives the brain the fastest and most forceful encounter with this chemical.

Due to the variety of ways to use cocaine, its users tend to span a vast spectrum of individuals and so its aliases are many. Some of the most common names are, "coke, white, snow, juice, crack, girl, etc." Along with its variety of names, come a number of interesting and peculiar articles that generally are instruments in its use. The powder form of cocaine typically is kept in small plastic or paper packets or baggies. One of the most often and easily overlooked means to transport the drug is in a folded piece of paper. Usually, this is accompanied by a short straw or tube of some kind used to "snort" with. Also, razors are used to chop it into a finer powder and separate it. Many times though people will use a card (i.e., drivers license, credit card, etc.) in place of a razor. If you are suspicious, it might be a good idea to look at, if possible, your loved one's plastic cards that are typically carried in their wallet/purse. If the cards show strange abnormal indentations in the middle of the card, this can be caused by crushing rocks into powder.

The individuals who smoke cocaine will usually possess a straight glass pipe with a piece of steel scouring pad compacted at one end. Since the "crack" is in a hardened form when heated with the flame from a lighter, it melts, producing the cocaine smoke. Some people use marijuana, corncob, or soda-can pipes with cigarette ashes instead of the glass and scouring pad method. Those who intravenously inject cocaine usually procure "insulin" syringes from local pharmacies. (Anyone [any age] can go in and buy these.) They frequently use a spoon or the bottom of a soda can as a means to mix the cocaine and water. Then, using a piece of cotton or cigarette filter, they draw the substance into the syringe to inject it. It is normal for these people to have teeth marks on the belts they wear around their waist. They use these belts to constrict the veins in the arm to make them more readily available for easy injection.

Since cocaine can be used in a multitude of ways, its users have varied physical symptoms. One of the most noticeable is paranoia. The use of cocaine invokes paranoia in the user. Medically, this has a great deal to do with the nature and power of the stimulant. Nevertheless, people under the influence of cocaine are generally paranoid. Cocaine has the unique effect of extreme euphoria followed immediately by emotional torture in the form of intense anxiety and the uncomfortable feeling of being very apprehensive. As a result of the drug having this effect, when non-users interact with those under the influence of the cocaine, they are frequently met with fits of rage, anger, and sometimes violence. This has a great deal to do with the internal emotional tension caused from the use. This effect intensifies depending on the extent of use and the number of days the person has gone without sleep. Because cocaine is a stimulant, users often stay awake for days on end. This opens the door of sleep deprivation. Sleep deprivation can cause hallucinations, paranoia, and other troubling effects. The longer humans go without sleep, the less rational they are capable of being. The human brain requires rest. Staying awake for days deprives the brain of rest, causing it not to function properly.

Cocaine addicts often keep themselves isolated in the bathroom since it is commonly the sanctuary of use. The pupils of cocaine users' eyes become significantly dilated (enlarged) while under the influence. Sometimes users will be found scavenging the carpet in search of "lost" cocaine particles. Along with methamphetamine users, cocaine addicts stay awake at night and sleep during the day. Many times you will find them doing behaviors uncharacteristic for them. For instance, your son who is a total slob, under the influence of cocaine, might be found cleaning his room extensively . . . in the middle of the night. Also, cocaine use in many people causes them to clench or gyrate their jaws. This is one of the side effects of the potent stimulant on the body.

Heroin

Heroin is the drug most people consider the "hardest" of the illicit drugs. Many view it as the pinnacle of addiction; meaning heroin addicts are the standard of what an "addict" is. This holds some validity, but is usually a comment made by a user of another substance trying to rationalize their behavior! Heroin is the antithesis of cocaine. It is mutually exclusive and diametrically opposed in relation to the effects of cocaine. Whereas cocaine is a powerful stimulant, heroin on the other hand, is a very powerful depressant. It affects the body in the opposite way as cocaine.

Heroin causes the functions of the body to slow. The drug affects specific neurological receptors in the brain (as do all chemicals). Its effect when described by users is "a warm, loving, euphoric, and peaceful experience." Heroin is an opiate. Morphine, which is commonly used in hospitals across the country, is a sister drug to heroin. Heroin happens to be its more potent relative. Heroin can be used in the same three ways as cocaine. Raw heroin is commonly called "tar" and literally is a tar-like substance. To snort heroin, it must be mixed or "cut" with a powder, the most common of which are sleeping aids because they enhance and do not detract from the effects of heroin. This latter method is the very form plaguing junior high schools presently under the name "cheese." In this case, heroin is being cut with Tylenol PM™ and put into capsules, which have been sold to junior high students for a mere two dollars a piece. If you are concerned that your loved one may be using cheese, be especially aware of the physical symptoms described further below (i.e., itching, runny nose, etc.) Also, the cheese capsules will appear in clear plastic capsules. The material inside will appear to be speckled and brown in color (the brown part being the heroin, the white or yellow powder being the "cut"). It also may be smoked; however, this is uncommon. Thirdly, heroin is also a water-soluble chemical that is frequently injected in the vein.

The items most often associated with heroin use are sleeping medications, capsules, plastic and paper baggies, syringes, razors, cards, spoons (black on bottom from heating with lighter), etc. Heroin users most often appear sleepy or lackadaisical. The pupils of users' eyes are primarily constricted under the influence and users tend to "itch" their nose and other extremities in an abnormal way. Heroin is much more difficult to detect from a behavioral standpoint than cocaine. Users who inject any drug will have "track" marks along the lines of different veins (i.e., inner arm, neck, legs, feet, hands, wrist, etc.). People who choose to sniff or snort either drug will characteristically have a runny nose or will constantly be "sniffing" abnormally. Also, they could possibly have red marks under their nostrils.

Methamphetamine

Methamphetamine is a synthetic stimulant that is not derived from nature. Cocaine comes from the coca plant, heroin comes from the poppy plant, but methamphetamine comes from the illegal "chef," "cook," otherwise known as the manufacturer. There are a variety of different "recipes" to concoct methamphetamines. Common ingredients include battery acid, farm fertilizers, mercury, elements of over-the-counter cold medications—the list goes on and on. As a result of its many various formulas for creation, it comes in many colors and consistencies. Some of these colors include (but are not limited to) brown, white, red, green, yellow, pink, etc.

Methamphetamines have many different names some of which are: speed, fast, meth, crystal, glass, ice, etc. Each unique batch of meth generally gets its own unique name coordinating it to the color of its substance. For instance, meth that has a green consistency might be called "kryptonite." Methamphetamines are currently plaguing our society because they are more affordable compared to cocaine. The substance is man-made, which makes it much more readily available to those who desire to partake of it. Consistently, its effects are very similar to cocaine. Meth, though, is much longer acting. Generally, it is less potent initially as far as "rush"—however, its effects last much longer, giving the user more "bang for the buck."

Frequently, it is in powder or crystal-like rock form. The primary methods of use are snorting, smoking, and/or injecting. Due to the toxic nature of the chemicals in its making, methamphetamines are extremely bad for the human body and brain. Little is really known about its long-term effects to the brain since different "batches" of meth differ in makeup. Meth has proven to destroy its users' teeth. Due to the inconsistency of its concoction and the toxic chemicals in its make up, meth causes many of its dependants to lose their teeth. Also, meth is notorious for acne and skin rashes. Resultantly, many methamphetamine users have lasting damage to their complexion.

A popular way of using meth is to smoke it. This is usually done in a glass pipe having a "ball" or "bulb" on the end. Some more non-conventional substitutes involve using light bulbs or foil "boats." When the meth is indirectly heated, it produces a smoke, which is inhaled. It is notable to mention that alcoholics who tend to normally pass out early are prone to using meth. The reason is because meth gives alcoholics the ability to overcome the effects of blacking out, passing out, and other uncomfortable effects of alcohol while at the same time allowing them to continue drinking for longer periods of time. Meth users' behavior resembles cocaine users' behavior. Users of this chemical are more prone to the effects of sleep deprivation because meth has a much longer-lasting effect. It is not uncommon for meth addicts to stay awake days and sometimes, even, weeks at a time. Paranoia is also very symptomatic of its use.

Marijuana

Marijuana has been deemed the "gateway" drug. Marijuana users are 90% more likely to try other drugs like cocaine and heroin than those who have never used marijuana. Marijuana is an herb. Formally, it comes from the *cannabis-sativa* plant. The "buds" of this plant contain a chemical called Tetra-Hydro-Cannabinol, better known as THC. This is the chemical that causes the euphoric effects in humans. Marijuana is a central nervous system depressant. Though not comparable in potency to heroin, it nevertheless is strong. Scientist have determined it is not physically addictive. However, thousands are "mentally" dependent on the drug. It does have some legitimate medicinal uses for patients in relieving the nausea of toxic chemicals required in treatment of terminal diseases.

Marijuana can be eaten or smoked. Usually, it is rolled into a cigarette referred to as a "joint." Other users prefer to smoke it through water pipes and various other creative smoking contraptions. College and high school age people alike are drawn to the innovative and trendy smoking paraphernalia that accompanies marijuana use. Marijuana is known by many different names such as, pot, weed, reefer, bud, smoke, ganja, wacky tobaky, spliff, spliffy, herb, etc. Sadly, our media has made a point to joke about marijuana, which has made it appear less detrimental. The truth is marijuana, just like any other drug, is extremely detrimental, maybe not initially, but definitely in the long run.

Any smoking paraphernalia can be used for marijuana. So virtually anything you can think of (and probably items you never would have dreamed of) are used by people to smoke marijuana. It is characteristic of the "pothead" culture to be highly creative in exhibition of their pot smoking. Red, bloodshot eyes are the most common symptom of use. Generally, smoking marijuana leaves the mouth feeling very dry; this is called "cotton mouth." Along with cottonmouth, users tend to feel hungry and are compelled to eat food; this is commonly referred to as "the munchies." Pot can affect different users in different ways. Some inexperienced users may not be able to function normally; however, most people can continue to function somewhat normally, making it difficult to know whether the user is "high" or not.

Weed (in my opinion) is very difficult to narrow down to "common behaviors." This is because most who smoke marijuana habitually don't exhibit a great deal of indicating behaviors except for isolation, being highly secretive, and stashing the drug and paraphernalia. Parents frequently misdiagnose marijuana use as depression, trouble with friends, and other non-drug related issues.

LSD

In the 60s, the Beatles wrote a hit song about LSD called "Lucy in the Sky with Diamonds." Not only did this song promote the use of LSD, otherwise known as Lysergic-Acid-Diethylamide, it encouraged a generation already embracing the drug-use movement. Acid is a chemical which, when taken by humans, causes among other things auditory and visual hallucinations. This drug, in my experience, is the most provocative to young people because it offers a tangible alter-reality experience. Many young people who are emotionally troubled seek escape and acid fits the bill. As harmless as this drug may seem little is known about its long-term effects. LSD is known by a multitude of different names such as "Lucy, trip, paper, acid, etc."

The actual substance of LSD is tricky to nail down. Generally it is a liquid. Pure acid has no color or odor. LSD is extremely potent. A few micro-grams ingested by a human can cause an "acid trip" (experience of use) for between 4–12 hours. Since it neither has smell, taste, or color, acid is extremely hard to catch users in possession of. The liquid LSD can be absorbed by paper and distributed on tiny squares of paper. These pieces of paper are usually referred to as "paper" or "trips." On the other hand, acid can be synthesized in a gel-type form, which can be distributed as pieces of gel, or in capsules. The possibilities are endless, which makes this drug very difficult to find.

Each user's experience can very significantly. Some users experience pleasant auditory and visual hallucinations, while, others experience horrifying results. Each "trip" has a great deal to do with each person's unique chemical make-up in their brain, and their emotional ability to differentiate between fantasy and reality. This (coupled with the fact that little is known about its long-term effects) leaves the use of LSD a very dangerous issue. LSD use could have prolonged mental effects into the distant future for each individual user. Pupil dilation is really the only noticeable physical effect of a person who is under the influence of LSD. Other than this physical symptom, acid has no other concrete ways to trace its use. In fact, LSD does not show up in a normal urine or blood screen test. This makes it even harder for family and parents to detect its use. Don't misunderstand. In some people, the use of acid would be obvious because of their mental awareness or lack thereof. So a user may exhibit, acting like a "space cadet." Other than strange behavior, there are few ways to look at an individual and know whether they are under the influence of acid.

Ecstasy

Ecstasy is classified as a "designer" drug. It's technical abbreviation and alias is MDMA. This drug is common in clubs around the United States and the world. This drug is man-made and frequently is "cut" or mixed with other drugs as a base to compress into pill forms. For instance, one could procure heroin-based ecstasy or speed-based ecstasy. Usually, this drug is compressed in a pill form with some creative imprint on it. Some pills will have designs impressed in them such as "four-leaf clovers" or the symbol of "Superman." Each batch is given a unique name and stamp to "market" the product. Many times MDMA is used in combination with other drugs, which multiplies its effect.

Ecstasy is uniquely known for causing minimal auditory and visual hallucinations, along with the feeling of floating or weightlessness. These effects make it the most widely accepted "party" or club drug. It enables the user to enjoy dancing at a whole different level. The most widely used combination of so-called "party drugs" is ecstasy and LSD. This mix referred to as "candy flipping" causes extreme visual and auditory hallucination coupled with the floating, weightless feeling. Ecstasy is very physically detrimental. Recent studies have shown ecstasy to cause irrevocable brain damage to the user. Also, when used while dancing, ecstasy causes the body temperature to elevate above normal. Temperatures of over 104° F in the body can cause permanent brain damage. Other times, users will "lock up." This is when, for periods of time, users will lose control of their body and fall to the floor in a locked-up type of convulsion, typically the individual will assume something like the "fetal" position.

Physical symptoms of a person under the influence of ecstasy are virtually the same as LSD. Again, dilation of the pupils is evident in the user. It is difficult to pinpoint those who are under the influence of this drug. Drugs like ecstasy reinforce the principle that parents and family must be involved in the lives of their loved one so they will notice all the signs of possible use.

Pharmaceutical Pills

There are multitudes of pharmaceutical drugs that are abused. For our study, we will look at two classes—the family of benzodiazepine drugs and prescription painkillers. These two groups of drugs (in my opinion) have the greatest and most significant potential for drug abuse. The first group is in a family called benzodiazepines. These drugs are central nervous system depressants. They are sold under different names in somewhat different consistencies and potencies; however, they all cause virtually the same effects in the user. This family of drugs is most widely prescribed for anxiety, depression, and nervous disorders.

The most common names of benzodiazepines are Valium®, Xanax®, and Adovan®. Please keep in mind these are their brand names and can come under many generic names. There are, of course, more drugs than these in the family and they are all just as addictive; however, the drugs listed above are the most common. Each of these drugs can be prescribed in a variety of dosages. Most young people who procure "benzo's" generally take them from family or friends' medicine cabinets. These drugs are usually readily available from parents who, sadly, are unaware of the potential abuse of these drugs. Many people in America are prescribed these drugs for legitimate disorders. Yet many people who desire to use the drug suddenly "develop" symptoms of anxiety to falsify the disorder in order to acquire the drugs.

Secondly, there are painkillers. These drugs are prescribed from a multitude of different doctors—ranging from the dentist to the family practitioner. Painkillers do just explicitly what they say: they inhibit the nerve and pain receptor cells causing a relief of physical pain. One of the most common side effect of any painkiller is that it causes "drowsiness, euphoria, etc."—giving it the potential for abuse. Many individuals who become injured wind up taking painkillers for the duration of their healing process. The problem occurs when they don't discontinue the use after their injury heals. During the injury recovery process, they develop a dependency both physically and mentally to the painkillers. Common examples of painkillers are Soma®, Hydrocodone®, Codeine® (same family as heroin and morphine), Diladid® (synthetic, pharmaceutical grade heroin), Oxycontin®, etc. To pursue further study of these drugs, I suggest contacting the National Institute on Drug Abuse.

6

Beyond Blaming

ONE OF the most difficult relational dynamics that arises within the addict's recovery process with those around him or her is the use of "blame." Sometimes this manifests from the propensity of people to find *fault*. That is to say, everyone wants to know "who is at fault" when addiction plagues a family. At times, in the case of divorced parents, it becomes easy for one parent to blame the child's addiction upon the parenting of the other. However, blame is something that can occur in virtually any relationship, whether husband and wife, parent and child, etc. The issue of contention is the detriment that is created by such behavior, not to mention the perpetuation of unhealthy dynamics within the family unit. Therefore, what is offered here is merely a sketch of some solutions to assist you in helping your family. Though this chapter is relatively short in regards to length, don't allow that to mislead you of its benefit to your relationship with the addict.

In this chapter, for simplicity we will use the term "parent," but if you are not the "parent" just replace the term with your role whether significant other, close family member, etc. We want to make sure each reader understands parents *do* have influence in the development of addictions. Parents do have further sway in the persistence of addictions. Yet, in *no* way can we establish that a parent is *at fault*. The project of attempting to attribute "fault" to someone in relation to addiction is nothing but a guise for a deeper sickness: *the blame game*.

It is my contention that blame is a tool used in tactical assault by addicts. Many addicts exercise it with precision in order to manipulate others. Below, I will highlight some of my own experience, though briefly, regarding the development of my own pattern of blaming. Hopefully, this account will bring to light the seriousness and far reaching implications of how blame can tear the very fabric of a relationship.

My parents divorced when I was seven years old. Even when I reflect upon this time in my life (and when you've seen as many counselors as I have, there has been a lot of reflecting) it doesn't stand out as a "bad" time in my life. Really, in all practicality for me, it was simply a corporate division yielding two isolated organizations which both had a vested interest in me, the only son. Though that articulation sounds someone cold and mechanical, it probably accurately describes my own perception of the events, which fell far short of the physical and emotional reality of the separation for my parents. This transpired during a time in history when it wasn't as common or socially acceptable to be a single mother with a child as it is at present. Soon after the separation, my father, for whatever reason, failed to fulfill the financial agreement my mom had accepted from him in the divorce. This financial burden along with the stress of working full time and not to mention the continued demands of motherhood put immense stress on my mother.

In situations such as ours, as is so common with broken families, the parent-child dynamic becomes blurred by life circumstances. One problem arose, namely, that this situation put me in a position to witness, probably with greater clarity than normal parent-child relations, the reality of my mother's mistakes. Not to say that most children don't notice their parent's mistakes, but in a single parent home it seems to be more enunciated. By "mistakes" I mean the living and learning processes that all humans take part in while on this journey called life. That is to say, I saw my mother date, have boyfriends, and attempt to have a social life. My mom, just like anyone else, got involved in relationships that spoiled. Since I was her son, her difficulties became my arsenal of personal information or "dirt," as some would say.

Here is the essence of what transpired: I saw her mistakes, then later down the road when I wanted something she wouldn't give me, or I wanted more *control* over her to make decisions concerning my circumstances, especially those she didn't agree with, I could use *blame* as a tool to manipulate. When she would advise me to make a positive decision or against a negative choice, I would, in essence, neutralize her influence, at least in my own mind, by using her past mistakes as justification to avoid taking her parental guidance and direction seriously.

Usually blame is inflicted from a person within your close sphere of influence. Many times blame is used to "play on" emotional "strings" stimulating you to react. Have you ever noticed that some people, especially parents and children, have the unique ability to cause each other, even the seemingly calmest one, to fly into a fit of rage? The reason seems to be based in the reality that those closest to you are aware of the chinks in your armor. Your children, family, and friends typically know your shortcomings. They know many of the financial mistakes you've made. They've lived with you day in and day out for years. They know all the intimate buttons to push. They know where it hurts. For this reason, blame can be one of the most detrimental behaviors a family can engage in.

Don't get the wrong idea. Parents, unfortunately, have a tendency to fall into this behavior. Some of the worst "blamers" are parents. They harp on past mistakes as if they were yesterday—when, in actuality, they have long since been dead issues. Sadly, this behavior can potentially stagnate recovery and growth for all persons involved. One should be avidly on guard to prevent it. Further, blame eats away at the moral fabric of any relationship. It is radically unhealthy, not to mention highly destructive. Relationships thrive on communication. Blame, however, perverts communication. It mangles truth while using it in a controlling way. It stands to reason that: *blame is a technique of control.*

So what we have when dealing with a person who is a "blamer" really is a person who lacks relational influence. Since they don't have the influence or control that they would like, they utilize blame in hopes of gaining ground by making others feel remorseful. It's essentially a play on the past. Blame is a personal attack at very least. This can really be one of the most painful emotional acts a loved one could carry out against you. The use of blame must be eliminated from any relationship to provide for the future health of that relationship. So how do you stop the blame game?

In the Case of the Parent

1. *Establish a boundary*—Times change and so do people. Humans, yourself included, whether young or old are continually growing emotionally and in maturity. Past decisions you have made are irrelevant in the present. That is to say, the past is just that, the past. It cannot be changed whether good or bad. Therefore, healthy relationships acknowledge the past while focusing on the solution in the present and future. Past mistakes you've made have no bearing on the present plight of your child. As the parent in the relationship, you are accountable to God, your morality, and in some sense the state. You can offer, but don't owe any explanations for your decisions. There is nothing you have to justify. Addicted persons love to play the blame game because it takes some of the focus off of them and their behavior.

2. *Let your behavior exemplify your counsel*—If you demand your child cease from judgment over past mistakes, you yourself must be willing to do the same. When a child blames a parent the natural reaction

is defensive. The defensive action is to blame right back. This becomes emotional "grenade-tossing," where both parties throw painful "blaming" grenades into each other's camp. Don't demand something that you're not willing to live up to. Which is to say, if you demand someone else quit the grenade tossing, you also must do the same.

3. *Disassociate the act from the actor*—It will take time for your child to realize their blaming doesn't affect you the way it used to. You need to pray and ask God to help you overcome the urge to fight back when the emotional grenades start flying. Your ability to not fight back will prove to be the weapon that will win the war. The easiest way to do this is to disassociate the act of *blaming* from the person. Many times, blaming is a technique that is subtly developed in one's character over time. It can even develop without the conscious awareness of the individual that they practice it. So attempt to think of it in terms of originating from someone's illness rather than a personal attack, though this is not an easy task to practice.

In the Case of the Family

Simply apply the above principles as they apply to your relationship with the addicted person. Remember always that blame fosters and justifies resentment. Also, it sets husband against wife, mother against father, and sister against brother. Don't let it draw a dividing line in your family. Blame causes unhealthy division; so determine today to eradicate it from all your dealings with your loved ones. You can overcome blame today and—*Recover All!*

7

Denial

DENIAL IS a devastating problem both to addicts and to their families. In essence, denial is a system of thought which denies a truth or group of truths. That is to say, denial is a cognitive defense mechanism that allows individuals to avoid facing certain realities, usually on the basis that such are emotionally painful. In completely reductionistic terms and for simplicity, the following example will at least move us in the direction of the task of this chapter, namely, to inform you of *denial* and its relationship to addiction. Hypothetically, let's say John eats pizza every night for dinner. His friend, Bob, frequently comes by in the evenings to hang out and shoot the breeze. One night, in the course of conversation, Bob comments, "John, you really eat a lot of pizza." John replies, "No, I don't."

You might be thinking. "Well, I guess it's a matter of perception." When, in fact, it is not. Here are the facts: John eats pizza every night. It doesn't take a degree in statistics to deduce that John has a pattern of behavior that is recurring. Now we are unable to reason, based on the information, the motive. This means, we can't say that John "likes" pizza. That information hasn't been given. However, Bob's comment to John *did* correspond to reality. John does eat a lot of pizza. John is denying the reality of his behavior.

At this point, we cannot grasp *why* John eats pizza every night or *why* John would choose to believe that his behavior is not more frequent than any other person's. What we do know is that John's perception of what is true is skewed. Bear in mind, John may function perfectly fine in the required tasks of each day. He holds a good job and takes care of all his responsibilities, despite his distorted self-appraisal. Now I know this example may seem theoretically ridiculous. Nevertheless, it embodies some fundamental issues regarding denial. Let's continue on in our example to better understand denial. Remember every thought/belief has an effect. What we choose to believe (whether true or false) determines how we act.

John could be ashamed of his habitual diet of pizza every night. If John is in fact "ashamed," then that logically brings up another interesting point. For John to be denying the truth because of shame, would also mean John within himself has determined his behavior is abnormal. There must be a cause for the shame. The cause for the shame is the inward conviction that "my behavior is not normal." This absurd example of John and Bob has far-reaching implications when dealing with real-life addicts. Addiction is a pattern of behavior usually involving a specific variable. For John, the variable was food. For others, the variable is illegal chemicals, sex, masturbation, pornography, lying, or alcohol. Amazingly, addiction can be as limited as one variable, such as the use of alcohol, or as complex as multiple variables.

Our example of John helped us to see denial in a practical way from the perspective of the addict. Don't get the idea, however, that the addict is the only one who usually is *in* denial. It is not without substantial precedence for the immediate family and those most closely related to the addict to be affected by denial, even to espouse denial themselves. No one is exempt from developing or exhibiting denial.

We have seen some elementary principles of denial as expressed by the "addicted person." Now what does denial look like when it is the family or friends of the addict? This form of denial falls under the subject of "enabling" as discussed more explicitly in a later chapter. It can be extremely detrimental to addicts in recovery if not addressed. Let's look at another case study: Jim is a twenty-year-old young man. He has recently graduated from high school and still lives at home with his grandmother, Betty. Betty has raised her grandson from the time he was sixteen, due to his mother's death. For the past two months, Jim has been staying out all night. When he does come in, he usually is perspiring as though he has been exercising. Accompanying this are Jim's dilated (enlarged) pupils, red eyes, and fits of anger. This is abnormal for Jim's character. Betty is worried about her grandson's welfare, and she tells her friend, Tonya, about Jim's behavior. When Tonya suggests the possibility that Jim has a problem with drugs, Betty adamantly denies the possibility of drugs. She is convinced that Jim's primary struggles are with his girlfriend and lack of proper sleep. Grandma, the loving parental figure, denies the signs of chemical usage in her grandson. Keep in mind, Grandma is the model. Her shoes can be filled by a mother, father, brother, sister, etc. The behavior in question again is denial. Grandma denies the evidence by dismissing it and assigning to it less-threatening causes. Again, denial is a *system* of thought. In our study we are searching for a practical hands-on understanding of the subject matter.

Why would Grandma, a nice, loving, and honest woman, deny what seems so obvious? Here is a practical theory: emotionally, humans have an almost natural pattern of resisting change. The thought of a drug problem causes every warning light on the emotional dashboard to light up. When the instruments signal a problem, the logical demand becomes: *Change . . . Change . . .* The response subconsciously is: *not possible, not happening, not an option.* For Grandma to even consider the thought of Jim having a drug problem would cause her to begin scrutinizing her own thinking and behavior. She would have to look at her own behavior first. If Jim does have a problem with drugs, Grandma's behavior has to change immediately and drastically. What is actually happening here at this stage is this: during the course of Grandma's life, she has subconsciously built "theoretical precepts" related to her impression of reality. They are ideas that Grandma has accepted as reality: paradigms.

Let's suppose that during Grandma's childhood, she developed the idea that alcoholics were bums and their plight was of their own making, namely, because they were unintelligent. Throughout her life she fostered, below the surface level, these ideas in her thinking processes. Therefore, she has a paradigm concerning the cause of alcoholism and a perception of the "type" of people upon whom problems of that sort attach themselves.

Now the facts about Jim's behavior come directly in opposition to her long-held system of "That can't happen to me." So, instead of releasing the false beliefs and being open to what in reality is transpiring, Grandma redirects the facts in an attempt to explain away the situation in a way that is less threatening. Systems of denial are analogous, in a sense, to the job descriptions of criminal defense attorneys. The job of a criminal defense attorney is really damage control. There are charges against the defendant. Whether or not the client is guilty, the attorney's job is to present the case in a different light to the jury, in order to get a more pleasing verdict. Even if the client is guilty, the attorney will attempt to focus on peripheral issues in order to direct attention away from the fundamental evidence. Denial attempts to redirect attention away from a sensitive area. The reasoning, logic, and choice of denial vary case to case.

A relative named Tonya, being a third-party, whose opinion is more objective, being one step removed, rather than subjective (in relative terms), seems to interpret the facts in a more balanced, realistic way. Just like any stranger on the street would realize, Tonya points out that the facts seem to point to the conclusion that a problem exists. Grandma is not emotionally prepared to admit there is a problem. Certainly, not a problem as serious as drugs. She defends her own emotions and behavior by rationalizing away the probability in her mind of Jim using drugs and justifying "the alternative" solution. The human psyche is a phenomenal machine. It is so advanced that scientists, have yet to discover all of its abilities. We do know, however, that the body has systems that physically sustain it, as well as emotion and noetic systems, which affect its daily operation. Within these systems, there are "defense" systems.

For instance, within the human body there is blood which carries vital oxygen and other molecules to the extremities of the body. The body is dependent on this system to live. Upon a closer investigation, we find that blood has, red and white blood cells. These cells, among other things, form a system of defense. When an alien substance infiltrates the blood, such as a bacteria or virus, these cells begin doing their job and fighting off the foreign substance. It seems our emotional and thought systems also have built in "defense" systems. Denial can most frequently be observed in the context of defense. It's a tool to deny reality, enabling the individual to continue in his or her present pattern of behavior.

What about the clinical definition of denial? We are going to use this definition to cross-examine our discussion of denial. With this information, we can be better-informed family and friends to those who are affected by addiction of any kind. The 2002 *Merriam-Webster Medical Dictionary* defines denial as "a psychological defense mechanism in which confrontation with a personal problem or with reality is avoided by denying the existence of the problem or reality."[1] Amazingly, this harmonized wonderfully with our present interpretation and applications.

Significance of Denial in Addiction

People who are in denial (within the context of an addicted relationship), whether parent, spouse, son, or friend can be highly detrimental to the overall recovery of the addicted individual. For instance, if an addicted teenager's parents are in denial about his probable drug abuses, there are a number of effects.

Effect one: Denial steals the focus of key family and friends while pointing their attention to peripheral issues. So while Johnnie is out snorting cocaine, Mom and Dad are home arguing about which girlfriend is the culprit of their beloved son's negative behavior. Peripheral issues, as used

1. Available from: http://dictionary.reference.com/medical.

here, merely refer to events, people, and circumstances outside of the primary issue. Thus, in a sense we mean distractions. They could be (but are not limited to) jobs, teachers, classes, co-workers, girlfriends/boyfriends, stress, etc.

Another vital area of importance is what I like to call "past issues." Under the umbrella of "past issues," we can hang depression, anxiety, physical abuse, abandonment, sexual abuse, learning disabilities, etc. Often, family and friends of the addicted tend to cling to these issues as the cause or problem of the addict. This is a distraction from the real problem. We certainly would never deny the probability of past issues affecting or influencing addiction, however, they are secondary issues to addiction. Both addicts and their enabling counterparts have a tendency to embrace past issues and focus on them, rather than the problem at hand, namely, addiction. This is distracting for all who are involved. If addiction is the issue, it takes precedence over any and all past issues. Until the addiction of the addict is confronted, the effort put forth in attempting to deal with past issues over time will be overshadowed by the addiction.

Effect two: Denial enables, that is, it assists the continuation of addiction. Parents especially, who are presently dealing with this circumstance, would jump in and say, "I'm not responsible for their behavior." Again, this issue will be addressed more explicitly in a later chapter. However, we need to be honest with ourselves. Whether we like it or not, our behavior affects others. Ultimately, we are responsible for how we affect others—whether it is for the good or bad.

Effect three: Denial prevents the addict from getting the needed help. This is one of the more basic effects of denial. I would liken my own personal addiction to heroin and cocaine, by way of analogy, to cancer (merely for this example). This cancer spread slowly and steadily to every avenue of my life. Addiction is a progressive illness. Much like cancer, the earlier it's treated, the better chance you have. Indeed, help is the object of this book. Without it, addiction is left to spiral madly out of control. Many are too prideful to seek help until it's too late. Asking for help can be a humbling thing. On the other hand, there are much greater and more tragic alternatives to asking for help. *Always ask for help.*

Insights from Life

In this insight, I will be telling you a true story from my work at a long-term drug treatment center. Of course, the real names of individuals have been changed to protect their privacy, but don't let that distract you from the accuracy and truth of the story. The characters involved in this depiction are Grandma and Sean. Sean's Grandma has been the sole custodian of him since his mom moved away in the pursuit of a relationship with a potential mate. Sean had a love/hate relationship with his grandma, but she, of course, adored her grandson. During this time, I was working as the admissions coordinator for the center.

Grandma was referred to us by the large church she attended, at which she had been a long-time upstanding member. Her initial phone contact with me seemed fairly typical. Sadly, as with most parental figures, she was completely oblivious to some of the "red flag" behaviors that her grandson was expressing. She was deeply concerned to convey to me that even though he had been using drugs, he was really "not" an addict. Her dear Sean, had been suffering with ADHD (attention deficit hyperactive disorder) most of his teenage and adult life. His drug history characterized the all too familiar habitual abuse of his prescribed medication for this disorder. It is noteworthy to insert here that ADHD is commonly treated with one of multiple forms of pharmaceutical grade amphetamines (speed).

He had commonly dismissed his misuse of medication by deferring the responsibility to his doctor's "inability" to prescribe the proper dosage for his "disorder." As I continued to probe Grandma's story, even more was revealed. She was very concerned about whether or not her grandson was actually an "addict." That term seemed a little extreme and probably impossible, according to her. "Certainly," she said, " My grandson isn't an addict." Next, she told me of his impending legal issues which revolved around drinking and driving. "Just once or twice," she said. As if everyone gets a DWI in his or her teenage years.

As should be obvious, this case, as become apparent in my own evaluation involved various levels of sickness, including that which his grandmother participated in. Hopefully, I reasoned, once we got him to treatment it would distance her enough that he might stop relying on her enabling. The main factor, though, was simply to get him into treatment. It needs to be said that all admissions usually have one major obstacle. *Nobody wants to go to treatment*, especially someone who is actively using. Usually, the addicts are never willing unless they have been beaten down by the addiction, drugs, the lifestyle, and legal system to the point of helplessness. This case was no different. Sean was *not*, under any circumstances, voluntarily going to treatment. For the record, I do not believe letting the addict make the decision in a case like this is the right way to do it. Even though legally you cannot physically force someone, I'm a firm believer that desperate times call for desperate measures. The ultimate goal is saving someone's life. So, strong-arming someone into treatment, at times, may be the only viable option.

Sean's strong opposition left his loving grandmother distraught. She couldn't imagine how we could get him the help he needed. Even though his behavior was very irrational and out of control, she still hesitated greatly in "forcing" him or "coercing" him to get the help he needed. This was my greatest struggle in the treatment industry: *getting the parents and family to muster up the courage to unwaveringly demand their loved one go to treatment at any cost.* This problem was the result of denial. Grandma, like many other family members in positions similar to hers, was in denial. Denial in this case can be deadly. Let's continue with our story.

Eventually, through much effort, we did get Sean into treatment. Usually, addicts, especially individuals who don't want to be in treatment (which is virtually all of them), begin manipulating as soon as they arrive. They attempt to manipulate the staff into believing that they really don't have a problem. They begin trying to manipulate the family by pleading and making promises that they really are done using *this* time. Sean's technique resembled my own to some degree. He knew Grandma was the "weak link." He knew she was easily influenced and coerced by him. So immediately, he began telling her how the treatment center was inconsistent. As you can imagine, this can be very persuasive. Sean, like most addicts, focused on everything around him, except himself and his problem!

In my experience this is *typical behavior* in virtually every addict that comes to treatment, some more than others. The triumph or tragedy of the addict's recovery usually rests on the family member being able to stand against the persuasion. Addicts have a keen ability to orchestrate, as if they were the directors, guiding life's actors around the grand stage. So Sean began his deceitful game. When clients in a drug treatment center stay emotionally sick for a long period of time, it tends to be very disappointing to those working in the clinical field. No matter how "professional" someone says they are, to be effective in the field you must genuinely love and have compassion for those you help—which makes this story so hard.

During the course of Sean's treatment, he consistently played on his grandmother's weakness, which was two-fold. First, she couldn't find it in herself to tell him "No!" and stick with it. Secondly, she didn't want to believe her grandson had become an "addict." As a result, for the first three months of his treatment he played games with the doctors trying to get more addictive medication. He did this by saying, "If the doctor would just give me (insert prescription drug name here), I would be okay!"

Any heroin addict on the street would be quick to tell you if his doctor would simply give him a prescription for excess daily morphine, he too would be healed and could live normally! This deception was the cement in the wall Sean was building between the treatment staff and his family. Eventually, Sean had fed his Grandmother enough partial truths, which biased her view of the treatment center's effectiveness, that she allowed him to come home short of completing the six-month program.

Today, Sean is in prison. He never really got clean and sober because we couldn't get Grandma to cooperate with the treatment team's recommendations and quit enabling her grandson. Sean broke his probation and picked up a few other alcohol related charges and then was convicted of prescription fraud, dealing in controlled substances for "ADHD." His Grandma's denial prevented Sean from getting the experience that treatment had to offer him.

Conclusion

It should be evident, merely by this brief sketch of my experience with Sean, that denial is an immense hindrance to the recovery of both the addict and their loved ones. Denial is difficult to pinpoint, especially in light of the genuine human difficulty with seeing our own part and behavior in light of our circumstances. Which is to say, when we espouse certain behaviors, especially those which lurk below the surface of our conscious behavior, it is hard to address them. Therefore, we must remain open to others who point these things out in our behavior. This is one of the most difficult aspects of treating chemical dependency, because we often struggle to see "our part" in detrimental or unhealthy social discourse. Thus, if for none other than the sake of the addict's recovery we must subject ourselves to being part of a community of recovering persons, whether addict or family, who are able to speak into each others lives and point out problematic areas that without assistance we might not notice or be able to prevent.

8

Rationalization and Manipulation

IN THIS chapter we will seek to swivel, as it were, the lens of our present study to bring two key issues into perspicuity, namely, rationalization and manipulation. These subject matters bear significant overlap both in meaning and manifestation in the addict.

Rationalization

As we delve further into the realm of addictive thought, we will now consider a commonly misunderstood concept: *Rationalization*. It is easy to confuse rationalization in the context of addiction with being rational in the general sense. In our culture, people are accused of "not being rational." "Rational" in this sense would mean displaying intellectual and emotional balance or thinking reasonably. One who is rational, along these lines, is one who is able to endure trying circumstances with a level head. However, this type of "being rational" is completely different from that which we are presently concerned with.

First, *Princeton University's WordNet 3.0* defines rationalization as "the cognitive process of making something seem consistent with or based on reason . . . [2] a defense mechanism by which your true motivation is concealed by explaining your actions and feelings in a way that is not threatening."[1] The second or latter sense is the one that captures the essence of rationalization, in so far as we are concerned with it here. Now we turn to develop the problem and a tentative solution to the phenomenon of rationalism in relation to addiction. Since we have established that addiction is a pattern of recurring behavior, which is sustained by its own protective thought processes. Rationalization, like denial, is another significant *protective* thought process. It is protective in the precise manner the definition articulated above states, namely, in that it enables the addict to conceal both motives, and of greatest importance here—behavior, behind the veil of explanation or rational. Thus, for the addict, who is

1. Available from: http://wordnet.princeton.edu.

constantly being questioned about various aspects of their lives, the necessity exists to acquire and employ reasonable responses that justify inappropriate behavior.

This is best expressed by way of example. Suppose that Johnnie is a 16-year-old high school student. He lives at home with his two parents. On Friday night, when Johnnie comes home from being out with friends at the football game, he smells of alcohol. Being the "alert" parent that she is, Johnnie's mother immediately confronts him about his apparent drinking. His mother, in a scolding voice questions, "John, you smell like alcohol. Have you been drinking? You know your father and I don't allow drinking." Slurring a little, Johnnie replies, "I don't know why you think drinking is such a big deal. Jeremy's parents let him drink beer at home. Why are you freaking out?" Johnnie has just exhibited a marvelous attempt at rationalizing his unacceptable behavior. We must understand rationalization is an attempt at making abnormal behavior, concepts, or thoughts appear *normal*. What Johnnie has effectively attempted to do is shift the attention from his inappropriate behavior to something else, eliminating the present focus on him.

Secondly, Johnnie subtly attempted to make his own crime seem acceptable and even reasonable by comparison to his peer. Notice the ease with which, if one weren't paying close attention, Johnnie may have successfully equalled the playing field as it were by positing "his friend." A few things must be said about this. First, one has to wonder if, in fact, Johnnie is telling the truth. Not in having the friend, which the parents may be acquainted with, but rather in whether or not his parents actually "let him drink." It is tempting to exaggerate the truth in different ways when one is seeking to rationalize their own behavior. On the other hand, my experience has proven both in my addiction and working in the field, that many parents, as hard as it may be to believe, actually permit their children to drink and sometimes even to use drugs. So your child, may be telling you the absolute truth when they argue that your rules aren't fair because so-and-so's parents let them drink, drug, or do whatever else. However, the point is that life and morality cannot be dictated by what "other" people do. For instance, many people cheat on their taxes, but when the Internal Revenue Service audits you, it won't matter that "your friend gets away with it." As a parent or loved one of an addict, it is your responsibility to maintain boundaries regardless of what others are permitted to do. There will *always* be some parent who will let their children do virtually anything and you must not allow what others do or don't do to cause you to back down in the fight for the life of your loved one. Furthermore, it is evident in the example above that his true motivation is to avoid the "threat" of punishment while attempting to overrule the "law of the land." If Johnnie is allowed to rationalize his wrong behavior effectively enough, he will overturn the rules that he is expected to follow.

Now let's explore another example of the rationalization process. Suppose that Bill is a banker. He has a beautiful wife and an extravagant house in the suburbs, filled with three wonderful kids. Bill is educated and affluent. One day he is approached by some business associates to embezzle money from the bank. His close friend is a vice-president of another bank just like Bill. He is embezzling money in order to get the new boat he's always longed for and to put his oldest daughter through college. Bill's wife has spent far beyond what their budget allowed on their credit cards for the past 10 years and the toll of interest and overspending was catching up with Bill's cash flow. Indeed, he had become desperate and was presently facing a terrible financial situation. In addition to the amount of accumulating debts which were growing daily, his oldest son is about to graduate high school and has plans to attend a very expensive university. His middle daughter is about to turn 16 and needs a car. Initially, when Bill is approached to embezzle money, he is totally opposed to the idea because he thinks it's just not right.

However, the more Bill thinks about it, the more tempting it is. Bill doesn't have a static source of morality, that is, he doesn't have a relationship with God, not the one espoused in the Bible who by nature is holy and just. "Times are changing," Bill thinks, "You just have to do what you've got to do, right?" It seems best to do whatever is necessary to help the family without the pain of sacrifice. Since ultimately, there is no heaven or hell in Bill's mind, he won't be accountable for his actions unless the authorities catch him. At present this seems improbable.

Since dishonesty can be rationalized by a man as a "necessary" act in some situations, Bill simply modifies his moral compass slightly to fit his circumstances. That, in turn, opens the door to Bill convincing himself that embezzlement is necessary; indeed, it is even justified. Finally, Bill succumbs to the pressure of the world and embezzles money from the bank. To his utter dismay, Bill is arrested within two months for money laundering, fraud, and embezzlement. He loses his wife, children, home, job, and everything he worked his entire life for. Bill rationalized his unjust behavior. Bill was able to rationalize his behavior because he was his own source of morality, the only problem—that morality wasn't static or righteous.

Here we have attempted to articulate, by way of allusion, what we hold to be important in the recovery process from rationalization, namely, a relationship with God. This is not merely an unrelated religious intrusion into this subject matter, but what should be obvious is that rationalization presupposes norms and mores as sociologists like to call them, or more simplistically *right and wrong*. Life's waters are difficult enough to navigate without addiction, but when trying to recover, the ability to make "right" decisions uphill against a mountain of past rationalization of unhealthy behavior can be quite a task—one which we contend necessitates a static source of morality; indeed, a static *moral person* with whom a relationship can bear fruit, namely, the fruit of acting justly and rightly in personal affairs. One way a person exhibits right behavior is by means of not rationalizing wrong behavior, but how is one to determine *right from wrong*? If right and wrong are found internally, then truth and morality are ultimately subjective. If that were true murder and rape could be justified as "true and right" to the individual who perpetrates those heinous crimes. Therefore, we contend that a relationship with God is very important to the recovery process. Can atheists get clean and sober? There is no doubt that atheists can and many times have gotten clean and stayed clean. However, we contend that God is necessary to successful recovery.

This has only been meant to serve as an entrance into the general contours, by way of hypothetical illustration, of the process of rationalization. Our point has been that in order to ground one against rationalization there must be a moral compass. That is, the necessity exists for boundaries by which an addict who has a pattern of distorting *right and wrong* can learn to rightly choose acceptable behaviors. Furthermore, rationalization, usually does not exist in a vacuum. Indeed, often it is expressed along with manipulation, which will become more lucid below.

Manipulation: The Art of Getting My Way

Building on what has already been established regarding rationalization, we move into the somewhat overlapping category of manipulation. In comparison to all other major topics in recovery, manipulation is by far the most intriguing. As stated above, illicit drug use is a generally unacceptable behavior to the majority of society. Even though it is becoming increasingly more socially acceptable, it is safe to maintain that presently it still falls in the category of social mores, meaning that drug use is not appropriate to the mainstream of our society.

As a result of society's view, drug users are left in a sticky situation. The user is participating in socially unacceptable behavior and must find a method to bridge the gap in cases where the information overlaps. What we are saying here is that when normal people learn that a user is using, the user must have intact a system of defense and subversion to sustain the continuity of their behavior. Whereas rationalization primarily happens in the realm of theory and thinking *internal* to the addict, manipulation, in our opinion, is a manifestion primarily *external* to the addict. That is, manipulation is concerned with *compelling others* to embrace what the addict has already rationalized. Therefore, we posit the question: "How does a user keep using if people around them don't approve and attempt to stop them?" The answer to this question is the key each addict develops to keep their addiction going.

The phenomenon of manipulation is best understood by analogy. Therefore, if one holds that life is like a stage. Upon the stage are many actors, which are people. Manipulation is the art of directing the actors on the stage of life for a prescribed outcome. The difficulty with this subject stems from the fact that manipulation in general can be both productive and counter-productive. It can be healthy or unhealthy. That leads us to the understanding that there are various kinds of manipulation, which are expressed in varying degrees. Since our spectrum again spans vast information, we must attempt to be precise. Precision would have us separate the kinds of manipulation and their fluctuating degrees.

As we have established, manipulation can be considered "good" or "bad." A good kind of manipulation would be characterized by a healthy communication exchange, causing the need to be satisfied or addressed without one individual exhibiting intellectual or emotional "control" over the other. To help us, let's think of a mother and daughter. Janice is the mother of Amy. Amy is a sixteen-year-old young woman. Her church group is sponsoring a lock-in. Amy is required by her youth leader to obtain a signed parental approval form and permission from her mother to attend. Healthy manipulation is simply Amy's ability to communicate her need effectively in hopes of coming to the desired result. Initially, this concept may appear somewhat trivial, however, it is not. In actuality, a healthy manipulation is required to sustain interpersonal relationships and could even at this stage be understood, in some sense, as communication—of needs. To further illustrate the "healthy" or non-destructive type of manipulation, think of the United States Federal Government. To sustain the government of the United States, the government requires each citizen to pay federal taxes. The federal government exercises control over its citizens by imposing a tax on them financially. Even though most Americans hate to pay taxes, few are willing to live without the government agencies and helps, which the taxes support.

There are sanctions or consequences imposed against and on those people who chose *not* to pay their taxes. Federal tax is not an option. Therefore, the government (to a degree) controls the individual through coercion. Since there are laws penalizing those who don't pay, the government effectively manipulates its people to pay taxes. There are many ironies in comparing the U.S. government/citizen economy and the family or friend/addict economy. Both scenarios embody dually effectual relationships. Both government and citizen co-exist individually and corporately. Each entity has methods of coercion/manipulation, benefits, and drawbacks for all involved. Through the manipulation of both sides, a desired result is reached.

As we are thinking along these lines, let's apply this concept to the family/friend and addict relationship. Generally speaking, the family's or friend's primary interest usually is the interpersonal relationship and general well being of the addict. Conversely, the addict's primary interest, though possibly coupled with the same, usually finds more focus around the orchestration and implementation of *using the family/friend to benefit the addiction and its demands,* whether they are financial, physical, or emotional. It is necessary that we understand at this point that in the case of addiction, this can be voluntary or involuntary in nature. At times, the addict in question will manipulate to get his or her way consciously while at other times, it might not be conscious from the standpoint that the action of manipulation has become a habit that goes unnoticed. Either way, it goes hand-in-hand with addiction and is part of the sickness that must be dealt with in order to recover.

Manipulation, in its most raw form, can be viewed as "conning." Most people are able to spot a con when it's a car salesman or a jewelry stand clerk in the mall. However, when the matter rises within one's close sphere of family or friends, it becomes a grievous task. Suddenly, our own emotions seem to prevent our idealistic view of reality. If you're a parent and you've been manipulated, you're not alone. I've spent the better part of my life manipulating my family. Sometimes, it even seems like a really unique ability. This ability today is an asset, but while I was in active addiction, it was a decisive factor preventing me from becoming healthy. Here is a an unfortunate truth I picked up in my addiction that I have seen addicts practice hundreds of times in their own circumstances. The best way to express it is simply: *if an addict can get their "way" in any given circumstance, then the addict has learned whether explicitly or implicitly that their behavior does not have to change.*

For instance, let's take some time now and travel through the lives of a few different clients that I have worked with to better understand the implications of real life manipulation. Addicts are masters of manipulation, as you will see. Keep at the forefront of your mind, as your read these stories, it is always easier to notice the problem from the outside looking in than it is from the inside looking out. Essentially, what will seem so obvious to you in reading these stories as terrible decisions don't always appear that way when the shoe is on the other foot, so to speak. The organization of the material adopted below will give you an overview of both addicts in active addiction (that is, ones who were presently using drugs) and addicts who were in treatment.

Examples from Active Addiction
Case 1

The following are true stories of individuals in active addiction though the names have been changed to protect the innocent and the not-so-innocent.

Bill was twenty-two years old. He graduated high school and attended community college for a time. Subsequently, he decided that he would rather get an apartment and work, as opposed to finishing his college education. Reluctantly, his parents went along with his wishes while advising him that it wasn't a good idea to quit school. Bill's parents were aware he had a tendency to drink too much. Even though they had raised him well and done their best to give him a strong work ethic, Bill remained an unmotivated and unfocused young man. During Bill's stint in college, he was completely financially dependant on his parents. They paid his insurance, food, car payment, tuition, books, and financed his social calendar. To say the least, Bill had a "good thing" going with that type of support.

His parents used their financial influence in his life to curb his drug use. They would sanction his funding when they would find out he was using drugs or drinking too much. It was very difficult for them, however, because Bill was in college and most kids his age were drinking and drugging socially. Finally, Bill moved into his own apartment. It appeared Bill was holding things together pretty well, for the first few months anyway. Slowly, Bill became more distant than normal. Whereas it was normal for him to frequently call and show up, suddenly, he didn't come home. Even though this seemed a little strange, his parents didn't view it as a major issue.

One day when Bill's dad came home from work, he found his tool shed in the back of the house had been broken into. Upon further investigation, he realized he was missing some very expensive tools and equipment. Very distraught, he called the police. After examining the scene, the police officer seemed adamant that whoever committed the crime knew what they were coming for when they stole the goods. Even though the logical conclusion was to question Bill, his parents decided just to file with homeowners insurance and let the matter die. Within a few days, Bill contacted his mother. He was somewhat distraught and sounded as if something were wrong. Of course, after this call, she began worrying about him and his well being.

Bill's communication over the next few days was surprisingly consistent and frequent. Then he dropped the bomb. While talking with his mother, he mentioned that he had been sick, which concerned her a great deal. Then he, in a round about way, let her know that since he had been sick and missed work, he couldn't afford groceries and rent for the month. His mother had always taken pride in making sure his needs were met. Bill had never gone hungry a day in his life. So her immediate reaction was to comfort him and let him know they would help him financially. Bill graciously accepted the help and seemed so sincere. In the following weeks other "out of the ordinary" situations befell Bill, sending him seeking the financial aid of his parents. Bill's apartment was broken into. Then his transmission went out. Then he needed money for doctor bills. Each time his parents would see him, they would give him the money he asked for. He looked as though he were sickly. It appeared he was losing weight, which concerned his father greatly.

Now there are some great lessons we can learn from Bill. What his parents weren't able to see was that Bill was strung out on crack cocaine. He had been fired from his job and hadn't paid his bills in two months. Over the course of the last few months, he sold most of his valuable possessions to acquire crack. Desperate, Bill even robbed his family's home to get money so he could stay high. It never started out this way. Initially, it was just a one-night thing. That one night however stretched into a five-day binge. Then Bill was a slave to the drug.

His desire for the drug even gave him reason enough to become a con man, devising witty and inventive schemes to secure the funds needed. He was a pawn in the hands of the master: cocaine. Yet he learned some things that would set the pattern for his behavior for years to come. Bill learned how to manipulate to meet his needs. Bill's addiction had advanced horrifically in a very short time. His methods also evolved. Now Bill would use manipulation in a powerful way to continue in his addiction.

You're probably asking, "Will Bill really continue this process for the extent of his addiction? How do you know?" These are both legitimate and astute questions. The answer to the first question is an unquestionable *yes*. Now let's validate answer one by answering question two. After a child learns how to walk independently, will he continue to walk upright? Yes. Why? *It works*. Children don't go back to crawling once they have fully developed their ability to walk. Once they learn it is good to walk because it works, they will continue in that behavior pattern. Addicts are the same way. Once an addict learns that manipulation accomplishes the desired result, it becomes a frequented path.

For instance, a bottle of shampoo has instructions. For clean hair simply: 1) massage a small amount of shampoo into hair until lather, then 2) Rinse and repeat. Now these two instructions are fairly explicit, right? No one would attempt to say that it takes a degree in engineering to wash your hair with shampoo. People do this all over the world every day. In fact, most of them know how to, so they don't even consciously think about the instructions. Why should an addict's logic be any more complex than this? In my years both being addicted myself and working with addicts, I have found that it is not. The cause is: Bill needs dope to feel better. Here is his process: Step 1) devise a lie and massage Mom with it until she hands over the cash, then 2) Use and repeat. Addicts all over the world do this every day. They don't even consciously think of the instructions. It has merely become second nature.

Case 2

Jack has been battling addiction for some time. His family is aware of it and supports his recovery. Last week, Jack admitted to his mother that he was an out-of-control heroin addict. He informed her that he daily was enslaved to serve the wicked overlord: heroin. Immediately, his mother devised a plan to get her son clean. She would move Jack out of his apartment and he would move in with her. She would take off work and stay home with him while he went through the horrific physical withdrawal. It seemed like a marvelous plan.

She was so pleased that he had been honest with her. Jack was her only son and she couldn't bear thinking about his life being ruined any further by drugs. So they packed all Jack's essentials and moved him home immediately to help him get clean. It was going to be a very rocky few days. Jack spent three days throwing up, shaking, and writhing in pain. During this time, his mother had enrolled him in an outpatient drug rehabilitation program. The location of the program was an hour from home, right over by where Jack had previously been living. So each evening after work, she would drive him an hour to the program, wait for him for three hours, and drive him home. To her, the sacrifice was well worth the reward, it seemed.

After about four days, Jack came to her distraught. He was very burdened and she could tell something was wrong. Whatever was wrong, he didn't want to tell her. After her probing for a few minutes, Jack confessed that some people were going to hurt him over $80 dollars he owed them. If he didn't pay these people, they would hunt him down. All Jack's mother wanted was for this drug nightmare to be over. So to ease the mind of her much-loved child she told him that they would take care of it tonight when they went to the treatment program. So Jack lined up the meeting to pay off the people, using his mother's cell phone on the ride over to treatment.

Following the outpatient program that night, they went to fulfill the obligation. These "people" met Jack and his mom in a restaurant parking lot off the highway. When they pulled up, Jack got out and went to the window. He handed the money inside and came back to his mother's car. Finally, everything had been taken care of. The nightmare was drawing to a close. After this description you may be wondering, "What about this episode was problematic?" What was it that happened? Jack used his mother's car to go pick up drugs, he used his mother's cell phone to call the drug dealer, and he even got his mother to finance it. Jack manipulated his mother to obtain the drugs he was desperately in need of. He didn't owe any money, he simply needed money. No one was going to hurt him. To the passerby it seems cruel and unjust, but to an addict, it's tragic yet necessary.

Case 3

During the course of John's cocaine addiction, his family attempted multiple times to get him into treatment. Each time they would get him into a program, he would break the rules and the program would "ask him to leave." This happened numerous times. His mother, desperate to get her son help, was running out of options. John had been asked to leave most of the well-known facilities. He even had been sent out of state several times. This wretched cycle had exhausted all of John's mother's strength. He had just gotten kicked out of the most recent program he was in and the family was at a loss as to what to do now. During the course of the day together, John seemed to be acting like something was physically wrong with him. Concerned, his mother asked him what the problem was. He told his mother he was having pain in his abdomen.

His mother had a difficult enough time trying to get her son the help he needed. She couldn't handle any more stress, so she demanded they go to the hospital and have it checked out. John reluctantly agreed. That day they spent nearly three hours in the waiting room. Finally they were taken to a room. Once the evaluation was done, John was asked to give a urine sample. So he complied and together he and his mother waited for the results. The doctor came in and by this time John's pain had grown severe. He was buckled over on the gurney, apparently in great pain.

The doctor seemed very concerned. John's urinalysis showed there was blood in his urine. The doctor advised them that he appeared to be passing a kidney stone. All of his symptoms seemed to be pointing to that. To help John with the pain, the doctor ordered he be given a shot of morphine to ease the pain and hopefully, he would pass the stone there at the hospital. John's mom relaxed in the chair in relief that there wasn't anything life threatening wrong with him. So the nurse came in and administered the medication. John appeared to feel relief from the tormenting pain in his body. The doctor then ordered a CAT scan to ensure that they weren't dealing with any more kidney stones and to see if they could track the progress of the one giving him such a great deal of pain presently.

A few hours passed and they took John to have the CAT procedure done. After some time, the doctor came back with a good report. He said there were no more kidney stones that appeared to be attempting to come out. He also said that the present stone must have already flushed the system because it couldn't be seen in the scan. It seems in this example that John is simply getting the medical attention he needed, right? Nothing could be further from the truth. You see, John had learned a tool of manipulation, at one of the more affluent treatment centers he went to, from an addict who was a medical doctor. This doctor taught John how to fake a kidney stone, because the normal procedure was to administer morphine immediately before running extensive tests.

John effectively manipulated his mother. You might be thinking this is an extreme case; nevertheless, it is a true story. This true story exemplifies a real mother's struggle with her drug-addicted son. This same type of manipulation can happen to any well-meaning parent under the right circumstances. As the family and friends of addicted persons, we must be wise to the devises of manipulation. We must be prepared to act rationally and sensibly in hopes that our discernment will in fact prevent misuse of our trust. When addicts manipulate, they not only abuse the trust of their loved ones, their disease progresses each time.

An Example While in Treatment

Tim entered drug treatment in April. Initially, on intake, he was desperate to find a program to get into because he had tested dirty on a urinalysis for probation. Since probation was involved, his options were slim to begin with. From the time of his admission, Tim maintained that he was not an addict and that he was actually just a dealer. He told the staff that his probation involved an aggravated incident in which he and his father, Jim, got into an altercation and his father shot him! Since most addicts have legal issues and crazy-sounding circumstances, this didn't seem that out of the ordinary in the context of an 80-bed residential treatment for men.

Jim owned a lucrative tile company and has had the long-standing habit of coming financially to the rescue of Tim. So, of course, Jim would be footing the bill for Tim's treatment. In fact, further investigation revealed that Jim was even paying for Tim's house and supporting his new girlfriend who had four children she brought into the relationship with Tim. So needless to say, Tim had his hands full with responsibilities and at that time had many good things to look forward to in recovery. Many people have a rough time initially adjusting to the climate of inpatient treatment, especially one with any spirituality. Sometimes they seek special treatment or "privileges," which is characteristic of addiction. All addicts seem to think that their case is "unique" and deserves special considerations when it comes to rules and privileges in treatment.

Tim, like many others, felt like the world revolved around him. At least that's the way he acted. From the very first day, he was reluctant to participate in the requirements of the program. He even got into an altercation with a client and physically assaulted him. After a few weeks, his behavior seemed to improve somewhat and he balanced out a little bit. However, he was still defiant about attending the required classes and activities. Then following a visit with his family on Sunday, he came into the office, sobbing. He genuinely looked as if he was distraught. He explained to the treatment staff that his father was sick with cancer and the tile business was in dire straights in his absence. Matters appeared bleak.

This treatment program stood out from most by working with "special" circumstances. However, it should be noted that this practice in the field of rehabilitation programs is unheard of. Tim made it clear that he couldn't bear the thought of his father being in this condition while watching his family's business go down the drain. The executive director of the program comforted him and began to devise a solution. He had to find a remedy that would appease probation and enable this man to be there for his father. So after serious deliberation, the director contacted Tim and gave him special permission to go home for a week on medical leave to compensate for Jim being in the hospital and arrange his personal affairs. Tim was planning to marry his girlfriend in the midst of all this commotion.

Tim was granted permission to go to one of the program's halfway houses and stay during the week. That would allow Tim to handle all of his business. Ironically, the director happened to be present at a banquet with all of the city and county probation departments that week. At the banquet, Tim's probation officer approached the director, asking questions about his treatment. The director had the intention of acquiring the approval of the probation officer in order to give Tim the special consideration he needed. This turned out to be a highly informative meeting. The director became shockingly aware of the other side to Tim's story. That day the probation officer spent about thirty minutes giving the director a synopsis of his experience with Tim. It turns out that Tim was on probation for assaulting his mother in a blind rage with a meat cleaver. In the midst of this incident, his father, Jim, shot him to protect his wife! Also, the probation officer was adamant that Tim had a history of dishonesty and manipulation to get his way. Then, the truth was revealed that Jim didn't even have cancer; he was in the hospital for kidney stones. Tim, who had been so convincing with the anxiety of his father's illness, didn't even go to the hospital once during the week he was granted! The reason his parents always went along with his story was because they were afraid of him.

This story is a testimony to the sickness and cunning ability of addicts and alcoholics to "work" the system to get what they want. Manipulation wasn't just a tactic for Tim; it was a way of life. Everyone connected with his life was a pawn in his mad scheme to arrange the pieces in his favor on the board game of life. Manipulation can manifest itself in many ways. This certainly is only one of many examples. Yet each case gives us practical insights into the deluded trickery of deceitful addicts. Pay close attention to each case. It is also notable to mention that each addict involved had devised a "justification" for their actions. Some were so deluded with falsities that their behavior seemed normal!

Protect Yourself

Hopefully, the above real-life stories have in some way comforted you if you've been similarly used, or have equipped you with some practical examples of what does occur when addicted persons manipulate the ones they love. Remember, if you have been manipulated, *you are not alone.* Some parents and family members become so ashamed that they don't deal with the issue. The people presented above were lied to, used and abused, and sadly, will continue to be until someone educates them to take a stand.

The key to understanding manipulation is to know that the root of manipulation deals with control. All the deception involved is pointed and necessary in the addict attaining his or her individual goal. This is part of the way many addicts rationalize their behavior. They disassociate their "person/character" from their behavior. They convince themselves that the deceptive behavior is "necessary" to accomplish the desired result. All of this rises and falls around control. Manipulation is derived from a person attempting to control a situation that, in actuality, is not under that person's control. Basically, it is a way to create influence in an area where one doesn't have any influence. Since most addicts are unable to consciously and justly influence those around them to help in the finance and procurement of drugs, they seek to establish another means of attaining their ends.

So how does a parent or family member combat manipulation? This can be especially tricky since most of the time there are emotional ties, which seem to mirage the one being manipulated by the manipulator. However, there are some essentials we can discuss here which should empower you to defend yourself from manipulation.

Separate the manipulation from the manipulator. We have to separate the actual act of manipulation from the person who is manipulating. In the context of addiction, manipulating is part of the overall sickness. Some may have been just as conniving before they became addicted, that still is irrelevant. The vast majority of people who manipulate their loved ones do so not because they want to hurt those they love. They do it in order to get what they want. Many times, they are unable to see beyond their immediate circumstances. Therefore, when we are able to separate the behavior from the individual, we then are in a position to deal specifically with the problem. This may be difficult, seeing as each case and its variables are different. Regardless, if we truly desire to help the situation and individual, we must not allow our own hurt feelings to prevent us from seeing that sick behavior is attributed to the sickness, not the carrier of the disease.

This in no way removes the addict's absolute responsibility for their personal behavior. It simply sets our sights on the problem so we can focus our attention on it. When we have successfully separated in our minds and hearts the behavior from the person, we are ready to move on to the next tool of defense.

Rationally process all the information and be slow to act. Addicted persons thrive in chaos. They seem to have a natural propensity to be "drama queens." Since the lifestyle is somewhat chaotic to begin with, it's not surprising that their interpersonal relationships are overflowing with dramatic affairs. Also, addiction in general has a certain mentality of "instant gratification" that goes along with it. It's simply the nature of the dependency. So our tactic to defend against being manipulated is *not* to allow the addicted person to pressure us into *impulsive decisions*. Most of the time manipulation is accompanied by pressure to act *right now*. This is one of the trademarks of manipulation. You see, the faster you make a decision, the less time you have to process all the facts rationally. This urgency can frequently be the difference between a good decision and a bad decision. Instead of reacting immediately (which that addict desires and often expects), we now must choose to defend ourselves from manipulation by refusing to make an immediate decision. Even the direst situations can wait. Many times the pressure is derived from those in the situation rather than the circumstances themselves. The slower you are to react, the less power the manipulator has over your decision.

Assemble a board of advisors to make all decisions. This technique I learned directly from my mentor Isiah Robertson, probably the most influential role model in my life. Think about this: every multi-million dollar corporation in the country is managed and directed by a board of directors. This ingenious idea prevents a totalitarian government in the company's affairs. It also relieves any single member from bearing the sole burden and responsibilities of decisions made. This same methodology can be applied to practical life, especially in recovery whether for the addict or in this case the family. Most successful people have a team, whether formal or informal, of people whom they use as a sounding board for their ideas.

This simple concept has revolutionized my life. Let me explain. In my own life, my addiction proved to leave me totally unable to make good choices for myself. So in my recovery, I began using people I trusted to give me their opinions concerning my ideas. They were able to help me see different sides of each situation that I, in my singular perspective, could not have seen. This alone proved extremely valuable in helping me to make the best possible decisions in every area of my life. This enabled me to see other perspectives than my own. To prevent from being manipulated, you need to assemble a "board of advisers." These people should be individuals you believe are trustworthy and reliable to give you excellent advice. Make sure you decide within yourself to allow these people to help you make decisions. Simply having them is irrelevant if you don't follow through and allow their influence to help you process matters.

Once you've gathered your board of advisors, *use them*. When the addicted person brings their drama to your doorstep and demands your action, take it to your board. This actually does three things. Number one, it satisfactorily *slows* down the immediate gratification of the addict's demands. Secondly, it provides ample opportunity to view the affair in the totality of its context seeing all possible solutions. Finally, it removes the sole responsibility. This fact alone can significantly help parents and families of addicts. Many times, addicts attempt to manipulate using "blame" techniques. This means that they use past situations (often portraying them in the light of you being the "bad guy") to try and influence the present. Since you and your board are making decisions now, no longer must you defend yourself solely on the basis of your own judgment. This makes the decisions even more unbiased!

We have now interacted significantly with both rationalization and manipulation. You should have sufficient armor to protect against the rationalization and manipulations of your loved one and their addiction. You should now be able to separate the offense from the offender, ease the pressure of immediate decisions, and obtain the good counsel of others while distributing the responsibility to a group rather than an individual. The sooner you apply these principles in your life, the sooner you can abide in the comfort and benefits of being a healthy family member or friend. Properly understanding addictive rationalization and manipulation will instill you with some of the wisdom to—*Recover All!*

9

The Hardest Word to Say: "No!"

LIFE IS full of difficult things for people to do. Some are physical tasks such as exercise, mountain climbing, or endurance running. Some are tedious tasks like the nightmare of filing yearly taxes. While yet others are difficult emotionally like a parent's death, divorce, or the adultery of a spouse. Of these latter difficulties, one stands out from the rest and is more universal to human experience, namely, a parent telling their child or a friend telling their close friend *no*. On its face this may seem quite simple. You might even think, "I don't have a problem saying no. I'll just say it and that's the end of that." But for many, doing just that is not so easy. In fact, working in a residential treatment center, I found time and time again that one of the greatest hurdles to overcome in the addictive family dynamic is for the family and friends to stop *enabling* the addict. Theoretically, it seems so effortless; yet in practicality, when the individual is in close relational proximity such as a child, brother, or husband, the actual practice of saying no and meaning it is a responsibility vast numbers of individuals are not prepared to do.

Really the heart of the matter is not so much the linguistic aspect, that is, simply verbalizing the word "no." Rather the difficulty lies in the fortitude one must find to stand strong in the face of addictive manipulation and pressure. So often family members say no, and yet when the addict is persistent, manipulative, and refuses to accept no as the answer, the family member finally buckles and gives in to the addict. Below, I will illustrate this by presenting the story of a young man whom I worked with. Again, what is offered below is a true story, though names and some events have been altered to protect the subject's identity. Here our subject's name was Jeremy. He came to our program on the advice of his lawyer. He was charged with his third DWI (Driving While Intoxicated) in less than two years. His drinking was out of control and the small town probation department in his county was pushing for jail time. Even though Jeremy's family was tremendously wealthy, they had grown weary of dealing with him.

He was exceptionally arrogant for a twenty-two-year old and his personality reeked of both insecurity and immaturity. He would without question be a "character" within the body of addicts in our program. From the moment he entered the program he expected special treatment. This was probably due to his family's wealth, he was well used to special treatment by the time we met him. Our facility was known for working with "special" clients and had no problem playing along with Jeremy's "needs." Other than his outstanding arrogance, Jeremy was a very likable fellow, as most addicts are. He had a unique ability to make people laugh. Soon I noticed that many clients in the program resented Jeremy, simply on the basis of his affluence. Of course, his egotistical rhetoric and sharp wit with others didn't help him either.

Having seen this phenomenon many times before, it became clear that Jeremy simply needed some attention. It was apparent that he had developed a dysfunctional system of attaining the attention he desired. So over the course of his treatment, I attempted to reach out to him. He was quite a unique individual, one prone to being excessively melodramatic, which made dealing with him intolerable for most of the staff; however, seeing largely my own reflection in his behavior I persisted and he responded well to my efforts. His family was generally pleased with his progress, and the prospect of his recovery was certainly looking good. That is not to say, he didn't make a daily effort to stir up dissention in the therapeutic community, but that is more or less normal. After about two months, be began pushing to be released. Our program standard was six months for the inpatient program.

Jeremy, being in his mind a "special" case, devised his own treatment plan that consisted of only sixty days. With great confidence he asserted both to the staff and his family that he was healed! *This is a very common phenomenon in long-term treatment.* First of all, no one wants to be in treatment for *six* months. Yet many times, circumstance necessitates this to be the case and in his case this was certainly warranted. Another aspect of the situation was the relationship which Jeremy had with his parents. He was an exceptionally demanding young man. Throughout his life, probably more so than most parents, they had given Jeremy virtually anything he wanted. Why wouldn't they, it was their desire, as with most parents, to give him every opportunity. Furthermore, their behavior of giving in to his every whim was largely developed as a result of parents genuinely being worn down over time. That is, as Jeremy became more and more difficult to deal with and ever more demanding, it soon became easier to give in to him rather than have to struggle against him.

Jeremy is a classic example of what in treatment lingo is called the "king baby" syndrome. Most families of an addict who evidences a "king baby" mentality don't have the means to give in to their every demand. Jeremy's family, however, did and this made Jeremy much worse than any that I had previously encountered. The treatment center hardly realized the battle that was brewing on the horizon. Within a matter of weeks, Jeremy had strategically set the pawns in place. He gave his parents the impression that the director had told him he was ready for release. He had made sure the treatment team was well aware that his parents were ready for him to come home. He told the staff how his parents thought he had "gotten well" and were ready for his release.

An inexperienced treatment staff member might be caught off guard by such an attempt to leave treatment. Virtually, all clients in long-term treatment endeavor, at some point, to weasel their way out of the program; it just goes with the territory of helping addicts. So when I became aware of Jeremy's slick plan, I made a phone call to his parents. It didn't take long to derail the work he had so laboriously produced. Yet, the events that would transpire following this could never have been imagined. Jeremy was very angry that his plan had been foiled. So he turned up the heat. He embarked on a telephone assault, targeting his loving parents.

Day after endless day, hour after hour, Jeremy would badger his mother to let him come home. He was so persistent that she became weak. Over time, he began to convince her, ever so slowly, that maybe coming home would be the better option. After a few weeks she softened to his request. The monotony and endless demands of her son left her gasping for air from all the pressure. Jeremy became totally consumed with the task. He abandoned all his responsibilities in the program to pursue his desire, that is, to get out of treatment early. The entire staff sadly watched as all Jeremy's progress receded in light of his new focus. His infatuation loomed as a terrible storm cloud over all the progress that he had achieved.

It wasn't long before the parents were pressuring the treatment center to release Jeremy simply in order to stop the incessant calling. You would think that people with such affluence would have the assertiveness to look in the face of their son, say no and actually mean it. Much to the staff's dismay, they were not able to do that and it would cost them everything they had invested. Reluctantly, the program gave in to the desires of the parents once we realized the parents had bought into his manipulation. We couldn't force them to do the right thing for their son. All we could do was "advise" and our advice wasn't heeded.

In the months that followed after Jeremy left the program, he acquired another DWI and was arrested two other times for alcohol-related incidents. Sadly, a really good kid with a genuinely bad addiction would have to pay a very steep price because of his parents' inability to say *no*. *You see, sometimes the addict (even though he or she is legally an adult) is unable to make adult decisions.* Please understand, Jeremy is always absolutely responsible for his own behavior; however, if Jeremy had been under these same delusions, but had a different mental illness such as schizophrenia, I suspect that his family would not have given a second thought to taking action regardless of whether Jeremy agreed or not.

If we truly love the person who has become addicted, we must *act*. Action frequently means saying no. This may seem like a passive action, but that is not the case. Saying no is our only offense. Addiction is maintained by a pattern of behavior that repeats itself and is sustained by a faulty system of reasoning. In order to address the reasoning system that is skewed, the addict's behavior must be stopped. Hence, with addiction *you cannot convince the addict to change their thinking prior to their behavior.* Which is to say, addicts need to be *stopped first* and then guided into right decision making. Or think of it this way: the legal system incarcerates serious offenders for two reasons. First, the objective is to hold the offender accountable for their behavior; and secondly, it is to prevent them from committing any further crime. The theory is that, sometime during this process, the thinking of the criminal will change. For addiction, one issue of primary importance is the latter, namely, preventing further damage (e.g. accumulating more criminal charges, car accidents, etc.).

Addicts stay addicted because they continue the behavior of using. This may encompass manipulation, lying, cheating, stealing, and anything else that is involved in the acquisition and use of drugs. The addict's "best thinking" results in their present despair. This might not make sense at first, but consider it for a moment. Some might respond to this by saying, "It wasn't my best thinking that got me here, it was my worst." This issue is semantic. No one has control over another's behavior. Each person, on a daily basis, makes the best decisions that they can, based on their reasoning. Anyone who denies this is just attempting to blame someone else for his or her actions. At the end of the day, whether good or bad, every person chooses his or her behavior.

We conclude addicts' past behavior has been a result of their best reasoning and judgment abilities. This makes it easy to see they are not capable of making healthy decisions for themselves. Consider this: What if your two-year-old daughter became fascinated with the razor you use to shave with? She noticed you using it and now that's all she wants to play with. You wouldn't have a problem telling her no, would you? Even if she fell down and threw a fit? What if she demanded the razor with tears in her eyes while using her most moving "sad" face? Any sensible parent would *not* allow this child to make her own decision about playing with the razor. Why? She is *unable* to judge what is safe. Her immature desires have clouded her ability to realize the risk. Perhaps she doesn't realize there is a risk because of her limited perspective.

Do you see the correlation? People in active addiction are unable to judge right and wrong in perspective. They have already presented enough evidence in their past behavior to show their shortcoming in rational decision-making. This is where the family member or parent becomes crucial in the recovery process. Unless the parents and family *stop* giving in to the whims of their addict, nothing will change. Why? If the addict's behavior continues to provide the desired result, there is absolutely no reason to change.

People who speed on the highway don't stop until they get a ticket. For some people, it takes further sanctions to get their attention. However, when they can no longer get the desired result without disastrous consequences, they will stop. So when you say no, on the front end it may be hard. Yet in the long run, you will be benefiting your loved one. Just to verify our findings, let's look at another case. Reagan is married with two children. He and his wife still live with Reagan's grandmother. In the last few years, Reagan acquired two assault charges and two felony possession of methamphetamine charges. These cases are serious business, especially since Reagan is only twenty-four. Collectively, he is facing a potential sentence of more than twenty years!

As any good lawyer would advise their client to do, Reagan was directed to check himself into a long-term treatment program. My first contact was with his grandmother. After being informed of her grandson's charges, we came to terms on the details and accepted Reagan into the program. He, like Jeremy, had a character of his own. Clearly, being raised in a rural area had significant import into his personality. It was evident from his first day with us that he had his Grandma wrapped around his finger. Our program was located about an hour outside of a major city, which benefited us by being in a sparsely-populated country atmosphere. This proved to be helpful for our clients, because it was removed from the temptation of the "city lights."

The abnormality was that Reagan's grandmother lived relatively close to our facility. This proved to be very discouraging to his recovery. Any time Reagan had a "special" need or whim, his grandmother would come to the rescue. This practice, even though it seems nice, is very distracting from the person's treatment. When treatment is comfortable, it ceases to treat. In no way are we advocating that successful recovery happens in an uncomfortable atmosphere, but some people's family (like Reagan's) contribute to the detriment of the client. Reagan was never able to learn how *not* to get his way. Any time the treatment staff adjusted his program to stimulate growth, he would be on the phone with Grandma immediately to remedy the situation.

Grandma would then rush down to the facility to ensure no one "mistreated" little Reagan. Not only did this disrupt other clients and cause them to resent Reagan, it also prevented him from growing. It would also prove, in time, to be the "monkey wrench" that would sabotage Reagan's entire recovery process and have far-reaching consequences in his future. Reagan fell in with some other clients who were not working a program. After conspiring, they devised a plan to bring drugs to the facility and get high. Their plan succeeded. Reagan even conned his grandmother into bringing him extra money, which he used to buy the narcotics. When the staff found out, as they ultimately always do, they confronted him with it. Reagan pleaded that it was really others who had influenced him; certainly he couldn't be held accountable.

Grandma was so blind-sided by Reagan's persuasion that she wasn't able to identify his sick behavior. Our facility gave him favor and did not eject him from the program, which unfortunately is protocol for most treatment centers without a second thought. Our program didn't give up on addicts so easily. Thus, he received consequences. Part of his consequences were for him to move bed assignments to a new room with a new roommate. Reagan, as with most addicts, resisted the change. He refused to move. This, of course, was not an option. So it wasn't long before Grandma was there to calm the situation. The program, however, was firm on their position. If he desired to be in our program and reap the benefits of our program's relations with the court system, he would have to conform. So he and Grandma concluded it was time for Reagan to come home.

After all, he had gotten a few months clean and against the advice of his lawyer, he left the program incomplete. It didn't take one month before Reagan was cooking methamphetamines again. Today he sits in a 6′ by 8′ cell, wondering how all this bad luck befell him. He still thinks it was a giant conspiracy against him that the system had singled him out. Grandma still goes along with anything Reagan wants to believe. The day he left, I personally spent two hours attempting to convince his Grandma not to approve and be "an accomplice" to sabotaging his treatment. All Reagan had to do was abide by our consequences and move bunks. We were willing to go to court with him and had a good chance of assisting him in getting probation and staying out of jail. Reagan didn't want to change. His Grandma didn't know how to say *no*. Today she writes letters to him in prison every few days because she refused to say *no*.

Don't wait until it's too late in your life. This tragic ending could have been avoided. Reagan might have actually matured. We will never know. Therefore, we must learn from these mistakes—learn to say *no*. It could save you a great deal of misery in the long run. Your story doesn't have to end like this.

How to Say No

Use a board of advisers to make decisions. If you have a group of people who are your team of advisors, this can relieve a great deal of the pressure in saying *no*. That way when the answer of *no* is decided upon, it will be at the reasoning of the group. In this case, it gives little recourse for others to blame you for decisions they don't agree with. Indeed, this process enables you to be strengthened by others, to reason rationally, and to have greater confidence on a number of fronts.

You must make the right decision even if it is unpopular with the addict. The addict shows him or herself to be incapable of employing sound reasoning abilities. This is evident from their *behavior*. Addicts always *say* the right thing, but a wise man once told me *"their actions speak so loud you need not hear their words!"* Others have expressed this by saying that the addict's "picker" (with reference to decision making) is broken. This illustrates the inability of the addict and alcoholic to "pick" or choose the appropriate option in any given circumstance. Just like in the case of the two-year-old child, you must do what is right, despite their present *unhappiness* with your choice.

There are situations you don't need to intervene in. Reagan's Grandma is a perfect example. There are times when you, as the parent or family, do *not* need to intervene on behalf of your loved one. This may be difficult for some of you because it has become part of "who you are." It is easy for a chemically-dependent person's family to embrace the role of "savior," or "protector," or "confidant." Sometimes we really enjoy being the one to take control and *fix* the situation.

Being a "fixer" can be just as bad as being an addict. To attain your own emotional health, you must not constantly be thinking about how *you can change their behavior*. Take note, one of the first rules of recovery is: *you can't fix them*. Once you adopt rule one, your loved one's recovery process will be well on its way. Your victory begins when *you* stop enabling. Learning how to say *no* will assure that you and your loved one—*Recover All!*

10

The Me, Myself, and I Syndrome

THE MOST baffling facet of addiction for parents and family is often the "me, myself, and I" syndrome. This, as you might have guessed, is not a clinical term or a medical condition. The "me, myself, and I" syndrome is the condition of utter inability on the part of chemically-dependent persons to see beyond themselves. Addiction is a disorder oozing with selfishness. This coupled with our societal bent toward avoiding pain at all costs and the mentality of getting something for nothing only perpetuate this faulty reasoning. Think for a moment about the society we live in. Generally, people expect to get skinny without working for it or to win the lottery rather than working hard and saving. My generation especially has been at the crux of a radical disjuncture between generations. Indeed, it is difficult for most today to conceive of life without a microwave, cell phone, and wireless internet access. These broad generalizations about culture are somewhat important to understanding part of the addictive dilemma. The microwave or "instant gratification" mentality breeds self-centeredness, which fosters the inherent belief that "the world revolves on an axis around me."

We all know someone (or many people) who is so pretentious that it is difficult to bear being around them. Many times, addicted persons become this way over time. This is due to the fact that addiction, at bottom, is a self-serving behavior. It is predicated upon "feeling" good now, regardless of how it affects those in the addict's path. This thinking can even continue into recovery, which makes for a very unpleasant sober person to be around. What is more devastating is the reality that, at times, loved ones inadvertently encourage this "syndrome." Parents/families/spouses have a tendency to *serve* the addicted person. Traditionally, this is known as enabling. On one hand, we all should desire to serve others and genuinely help them. However, often this assistance, in time, and especially when addiction enters the picture soon becomes unhealthy. Usually, those who enable the addict are unaware of ways in which they contribute to the illness and even have trouble taking it seriously when others point that behavior out. Indeed, sometimes the family member in an effort to cope with the addict develops this tendency, which is a difficult habit to break.

Since addiction by nature is so selfish, anything that contributes to self-seeking behavior is negative for the addict.

The Game

To help in illuminating this subject, it's necessary for us to survey a real person's life and struggles to get clean and sober. Hopefully, his shortcomings and mistakes can help us learn about this damaging condition of self-infatuation. Meet Doug. Doug is a 28-year-old man. He had struggled with heroin and cocaine extensively for a number of years. At one time, he was involved in the stock market, making upwards of one hundred and fifty to two hundred thousand dollars a year. Unquestionably, he was highly intelligent and generally a pleasant person to be around. He was raised in a Christian home and had a supportive family.

Doug's incredible aptitude to generate revenue, win friends, and influence people have contributed to an inflated self-image and personal overconfidence. Generally, however, it needs to be said that Doug is a good-hearted person. It was relatively obvious that he typically meant well. When it came to inpatient treatment, Doug fared well. That is, he had been to multiple programs and therefore, understood what was expected, knew the right things to say and so forth. From that standpoint he always appeared to progress well, each time we saw him. The one setback to associating with Doug was his unique ability to think only about himself. Even in the midst of conversation among his friends, it became obvious to the observer that he always seemed to move conversations, subtly, toward himself and his desires. Furthermore, his Christian background enabled him to employ the "right" rhetoric to appear to be growing spiritually, especially to his counselors.

He made it through inpatient treatment and moved into a half-way house. There he pursued a career as a physical trainer. This was a new field for him with a whole world of opportunities. Immediately, he found success. Success, however, was not new to him because he always possessed the unique ability to perform well and therefore, to exceed expectations. So within a short period of time, he gained corporate attention by leading his store in sales. This of course, offered him significantly greater financial opportunities. Indeed, along with his success, he foud himself in a relationship with what he believed to be a great girl. During the course of all his success, however, somehow he began to slip in the arena of recovery.

For a time, he concealed it, very well. He was able to hold his head above water enough that nobody noticed, for a while.

As his relationship with the woman progressed, it became more apparent to those he lived with that he would be pursuing more seriously the relationship and ultimately moving out of the half-way house. During this time, he began using again. At first he just stuck his toe in the water again. It seems his success gave him an over-confidence. He thought he could drink socially without going back to the drugs. He was wrong. Soon he moved out of the half-way house into his own place. His parents, in hopes of assisting him, decided to sign the lease for him. They also paid for the apartment a year in advance to help him get on his feet. Though he had the apartment, he began living with his girlfriend. So he sub-let the apartment out, taking the revenue from it into his pocket.

He also somehow convinced his girlfriend to help him "pay" rent for the apartment. (She wasn't aware it was paid for.) During this time, his income from his own employment was exceeding four thousand dollars a month. While generating all this income, his addiction was festering out of control. It wasn't long before Doug pulled down his towering accomplishments around him. Sadly, his charisma couldn't support his character and recovery. So intervention was again necessary and he was given more treatment. When his deception was exposed, he was still oblivious to the depth of his dishonesty. He viewed the whole problem as simply a "setback." He didn't take it seriously.

Doug wouldn't dare look inward at the truth. His thinking was so ingrained in self-fulfillment, self-acquisition, and success that it remained impossible for him to think anything could possibly be "*wrong*" with him or his character. So Doug began building his life again. Sure he had messed up, but at this point, it hadn't gotten far enough to do excessive damage. Within a short time, he had regained all that he put at risk. He got back the job, the money, the woman, and all the toys that went along with that. Driven to come back from his setback, he set his heart again to succeed. It didn't take long, a few months, and he was back on top. Or so it appeared.

Then suddenly and in the perception of most, he disappeared. Gone in a plume of smoke, he vanished. To those who knew the pattern of addiction, it was clear where he was, but for others in his life, they had no clue. He was using again. Days went by and still no sign of him. When he reappeared chaos ensued. This time he had sold his girlfriend's car to the dope man. He robbed, cheated, and stole as much cash as he could get his hands on and the dope still had him. This time was worse than before.

He was found hiding at a local motel. His bridges again had been burned and crack cocaine had stolen the success he had achieved right out from under him.

On his way back to treatment, after selling his girlfriend's car, stealing money from her, disappointing his parents, family, and friends, stealing money from a different girlfriend, and abandoning his job, his primary concern was how long he would have to stay in the program *this time*! Amazing, isn't it? In the midst of such destruction, after hurting everyone close to him, all he could think about was himself. Doug is not alone. This is a trademark of addiction.

Doug was consumed with "me, myself, and I." Self-infatuation is the rudimentary principle sustaining addiction. It was this cause that blindsided Doug from effectively addressing his issues and developing a successful program of long-term recovery. His intelligence and ability caused him to over estimate his recovery process. Intelligence and ability can never (in themselves) sustain long-term sobriety. Sobriety is maintained by emotionally, psychologically, and physically healthy systems of living that are applied one day at a time. Also, in my own experience—service, that is, the process of helping others is the best way for an addict to "get out of themselves" and break away from self-centeredness in the extreme. If a person consumes all of their thoughts in regard to themselves they have little desire to help others.

The mentality of "me, myself, and I" goes hand-in-hand with the drug/alcohol culture. In the drug world, it's the only way to live. Indeed, it is the only way to survive in such a chaotic world of illicit trade. Nobody in that world looks out for the safety, well-being, or happiness of others. To compensate for this, people start to look out for themselves only. Life becomes a game of acquiring possessions and conquering all things and people which oppose self-gratification. This system of thought, however, easily becomes habit. If unnoticed, it can subtly creep even into recovery. Selfishness can quickly erode the emerging fruit in a budding recovery program. What makes it even more difficult is when the selfish person is ignorant of their own self-seeking behavior, which is frequently the case.

This same behavior may not appear in the actions of your loved one as expressly as they did in Doug's case. Selfishness hides in the shadows, a veiled adversary existing below the surface. It looms behind one's speech and in the recesses of one's consciousness. Therefore, it must be taken seriously, especially when addiction is brought into the picture. The ability of the family to perceive and guard against the wiles of an addict's selfishness can be the difference between life and death. So you may be asking,

"How can I help my loved one who is selfish and utterly consumed with themselves?" As with alcoholism, there is no instant fix. So if you are looking for an overnight cure, it won't be found here. There are a few healthy responses you can exhibit in hopes that it would draw your loved one to grow out of selfishness.

The first thing you can do is begin your own recovery. Before you can positively impact the addict's life, you must first take personal inventory. Begin by asking yourself in what ways you are selfish. All people are selfish to a degree and in specific matters. On the basis that it is difficult to help someone else before being in touch with oneself, I encourage you here to be searching, fearlessly and honestly, to admit your own selfishness. Make a decision to work on this and at very least to be more conscious of it. This, in turn, will help you to be prepared to operate in a relationally healthy way toward the addict with whom you are concerned. Further, ask yourself how your own personal behavior facilitates their selfishness. Once you have determined some key areas in which *you* aid the persistence of their selfishness, make a resolve to cease from these behaviors. Your willingness to grow emotionally will both serve as a model to the addict as well as open their minds to listen to you on the basis of your willingness to grow.

Next, watch and listen. Now that you've been equipped with the information about the destructive nature of selfishness, spend some time actually listening and watching the addict's words and behavior. Quietly, note the areas they are most selfish in. Even if their sole consideration is themselves, still see if you can pin-point areas in which they are excessively selfish. Once you appreciate the environment you are in, only then can you make an effort to change the situation.

Develop a plan. With your newly found results, come up with a strategy to help illuminate your loved one's selfishness to them. Sometimes the simple awareness will help in alleviating selfishness. Other times, it takes more extreme measures. Be prepared to be patient. Growing out of selfishness can take time.

11

Is There Help?

AFTER A parent/family has come to grips with the actuality of their loved one's probable addiction, a truly perplexing and desperate question arises: "Is there help out there?" As if the realization that their loved one has a life-threatening illness and is in need of immediate treatment wasn't enough, they are now plummeted into the confusing sphere of treatment and counseling program options. Rehabilitation in recent years has become a multi-billion dollar business, which has had both positive and negative effects. Positively, there are now many channels through which addicts and their families can get help. Conversely, the task of assessing the seriousness of the problem and choosing the *right* program has become a matter of real difficulty. What types of programs are available? What essentials should I look for in selecting a recovery program?

In this section, we hope to bring clarity to these and many other questions. These decisions can mean the difference between the life and death of the addict. Finding the right treatment or counseling program is not like getting an oil change. No matter where you go, you do not get the same job done. Remember, we are dealing with human lives, not cars. Unfortunately, people tend to choose programs based on amenities and accessories. This tactic might be a great way to shop for apartments or automobiles, but it doesn't work for finding the right help for recovery. There is no exhaustive guide to these questions either. Someone must have forgotten to write, "Getting Your Kid into Rehab for Dummies!" However, what is offered here is a step in that direction.

At the outset it is first necessary to understand how to evaluate the addict's need in light of the options available. In this matter, there are "degrees" or levels of treatment, which cater to the diversity in addicts and their addictions. Sometimes long-term treatment isn't necessary, other times it is the only reasonable solution. Where is the line drawn? How can someone determine what the addict needs?

Options Available

First, we must define the difference in rehabilitation solutions. The primary divisions in types of drug and alcohol recovery solutions are inpatient and outpatient programs. These terms are relatively self-explanatory, in so far as they designate the location of the patient in regards to the program, namely, inpatient means that the patient *lives* at the program facility, whereas the converse is true of outpatient. However, they can be confusing so we will look at each individually. Regarding inpatient programs, they usually provide a hospital-like environment. Some inpatient programs are located inside hospitals. Others are self-sustaining, stand-alone facilities, often analogous in design to a retirement home. They hope to model a mediate position between a "sterile" hospital environment and a warm home-like environment for the addict. Most inpatient programs are staffed with licensed medical nurses, counselors, and doctors. Even though many do have licensed medical staff, some do not. This does not necessarily make them "less" of or "less quality" program. My life was radically changed in long-term inpatient program that did not formally employ a medical staff, but they outsourced their medical/clinical care.

Furthermore, inpatient programs are designed to facilitate community living. That is, the community model is held in high regard for the purpose of learning to "live again" with others in a similar situation. This model provides for the addict to be removed from their using environment and placed in a safe and secure atmosphere that can foster their development. Living with other addicts is extremely beneficial to the recovery of individuals for a number of reasons. Probably the greatest reason is to enable the addict to get objective feedback on their behavior and attitude. Often we don't "hear" hard truths from those closest to us, such as family members, for any number of reasons. The inpatient dynamic also pushes the addict to adapt to change and social integration, both issues that do not come naturally to an addict in early recovery. The inpatient model is able, in a controlled environment, to give the addict the ability to learn to function in daily, routine activities while attending both individual and group counseling/therapy.

Usually, these programs offer a more rigorous and challenging recovery curriculum than other options available while providing the patients with a unique, healthy atmosphere. Typically, the patients are not permitted to leave the facility prior to completion, unless they opt out of the program. This helps to keep those who are in the program chemical-free while in treatment. Of course, it has its negatives as well, in that, eventually it is necessary for an addict to be adapted *back into* his or her home environment. Further, this model alleviates, to a degree, the temptations to drink or use more than any other mode of rehabilitation.

The vast majority of inpatient rehabilitation programs last a maximum of 30 days. Unfortunately, this is not optimal; the reason for this practice is based on the fact that most insurance providers which *do* cover drug/alcohol treatment (which is few) generally will not pay for treatment longer than 30 days. There are some inpatient programs whose curriculum is 60, 90, or 180 days. These programs, however, are few and far between. Nevertheless, *it has been my experience that thirty-day programs often are not long enough for lasting change. Therefore, I strongly encourage long-term treatment.*

The next type of treatment to be considered is outpatient. Outpatient programs allow the patient to continue living at home and working at their normal jobs. The patients in these programs attend classes and both individual and group counseling at the recovery center, but continue to live in their home environment. There are varying degrees of outpatient care. For instance, there is what is considered "intensive" outpatient, which typically is day treatment. That is, the patients spend about eight hours a day at the treatment program attending classes, while working with counselors and therapists everyday for an extended period of time. Obviously, this option requires a greater time and financial demand since the addict could not continue to work a normal job. Other than "intensive" outpatient programs simply vary to a lesser degree in the number of hours during the day which is required. Some of these consist of either exclusively morning or evening sessions.

Outpatient programs provide structure though to a significantly lesser degree than inpatient programs. The great value these programs have is found in their unique ability to provide assistance to addicts who are able to continue in their profession. This option is only viable in the case that the addict is *able* to do so, which more often than not simply isn't the case. Another downside to outpatient programs lies in the freedom that is granted to the addict. When dealing with addicts and alcoholics, it is rare that of their own accord they be able to stop using chemicals for even the duration of a few weeks for the outpatient program. More serious alcoholics and addicts may not be able to handle the freedom of continuing to live in their normal environment that has enabled them to use chemicals. These latter considerations must always be weighed when selecting a program right for your situation.

Both inpatient and outpatient programs are beneficial, as long as it is understood, they tend to cater to two types of addicts, the former for the most progressive manifestations of addiction and the latter for earlier and preemptive cases. Each individual's case must be evaluated to determine the needed treatment.

Outside of inpatient and outpatient rehabilitation programs, there exists a diversity of options. Four major types will be addressed here: individual counseling, group counseling programs, Alcoholics Anonymous/Narcotics Anonymous groups, and Overcomer groups. These groups comprise the majority of options outside formal treatment (inpatient/outpatient). The first of our four is individual counseling. While individual counseling can be prescribed for multitudes of issues, our focus is drug and alcohol counseling. There are many advantages and few disadvantages to individual counseling. The degree of success with it will be determined by the severity of the addiction and the *honesty* of the patient.

The nature of addiction tends to be highly secretive. Since using chemicals is typically frowned upon, those who do use generally hide it. One result of this "secretive" behavior is that the chemically-dependent person stops communicating their feelings. They also tend to appreciate others advice and direction much less, if at all. Counseling provides an excellent opportunity for the addict to establish a healthy interpersonal relationship outside the sphere of using. It provides ample opportunity to become honest with someone who assuredly will hold the information confidential. The lifestyle of a drug/alcohol user is one lacking trust. Most people who use drugs lie, cheat, and steal to support their habit. Especially, within the ranks of addiction there is little (if any) trust. Counseling helps the addict to regain trust in others as well as a multitude of other healthy relational skills.

Conversely, individual counseling also has the potential to become unhealthy, especially the more manipulative the client. This would generally take place in the case of an individual who is dishonest with the counselor. The counselor's only interaction in this scenario is once a week or so at an office visit. If the patient is deceptive and dishonest with the counselor, they will be unable to give the best counsel or address all of the issues. Many addicts must be held accountable in a controlled environment since addiction is a deceptive disorder.

The problem is that the addict goes to counseling and makes everything appear well, when, in fact, his or her report is false. When the addict's real life is out of control and their use is spiraling madly, it is not uncommon for their story to the counselor is "My life is going well." Granted counselors are practicing professionals who are well equipped to deal with this, there is still a potential for abuse which should be guarded against. Conversely, counseling generally helps those who are willing and honest. What is more, seeing the correct *type* of counselor is probably the most vital issue. Just any counselor is not advised in situations regarding addiction, rather, specifically seek out an LCDC (Licensed Chemical Dependency Counselor) and/or an LPC (Licensed Professional Counselor).

The second type of recovery option is a group-counseling program. These are usually weekly classes put on by licensed professional counselors. Sometimes these type groups are affiliated with in or outpatient chemical dependency programs. It should be noted that you might encounter certain groups designed and marketed to "offenders." Similar to the phenomenon of "Defensive Driving Schools" which help you avoid a speeding ticket going on your record, these special interest groups target offenders, such as those who were arrested with DWI (Driving While Intoxicated) charges. Courts frequently require certain group therapies and classes in that regard. So be aware of what is available and be cautious to investigate the program assisting your loved one to join. These programs can be very effective when prescribed to the right person. As with any of the treatment options discussed here, the success rate is usually based on the individual's desire, effort, and commitment. Programs such as these usually provide an above average menu of addictive education. The downside is that they offer limited accountability.

Alcoholics Anonymous/Narcotics Anonymous are exceptional programs assisting the chemically dependent to recover. These programs are virtually identical in many regards and completely distinct in others. However, for our purposes here both may be seen as equal in value and productivity for addiction/alcoholism. Also, contrary to popular opinion, addicts can, in my estimation, achieve sobriety in either program as can alcoholics. They both are founded upon a a 12-step structure and support network. Virtually all inpatient/outpatient treatment programs teach the 12-Steps of A.A., N.A. or both. Also, programs strongly advise their patients to become regular members of either group.

The chief reason that A.A./N.A. is so highly recommended is because both programs provide structured steps for living, meetings, and social activities. These areas are essential to long-term recovery. Millions of people have recovered and continue to maintain their recovery in these twelve-step programs. The twelve-steps require the person to look within themselves rather than pointing the finger at others. They also encourage the person to become spiritual and at least be consciously aware of the spiritual aspects of addiction/alcoholism. For a moment, we must address a major problem predominately in American churches. Since the A.A./ N.A. program does not specifically promote Christianity, it has been, by some American pastors and church members, condemned. This is tragic. While A.A./N.A. does not expressly promote Christianity, the issue is that it promotes recovery and spirituality. Don't allow someone else's opinion to sway the vital opportunity your loved one has to recover through the help found in these programs merely on the basis that "it is not a Christian program."

A.A./N.A. meetings are not meant to be religious or necessarily a source of spirituality. Most people lose sight of this. Church, distinctly, is meant to learn about God. A.A./N.A. is distinctly meant to be a group of people helping each other to stay clean and sober. Regardless of what anyone tells you, I have met many good Christian people in A.A./N.A. and they are there to stay clean and sober, not necessarily to be religious.

An "Overcomer" group is simply the exclusively Christian version of the A.A./N.A. program. This program has twelve steps as well. All of which read virtually identically to the A.A./N.A. program exchanging the words "higher power" in A.A./N.A. for the name of Jesus Christ. This program is very helpful in many ways. However, there are a few downsides to it. The first is simply that the Overcomers program has not been around for the last fifty or so years. There are not Overcomer meetings in every city. With less government, these groups are easier prey for leaders who want to dominate and control the administration of the group. Also, these groups (more often than not) are somewhat judgmental of A.A. and have a tendency to, in their attempt to *stay distinctly* Christian, over-spiritualize matters, which can be detrimental.

Twelve-step programs as a whole have impacted the field of recovery in a more powerful and long-lasting way than any other program. They provide a pattern for living. They encourage the "mentoring" concept. Also, they foster healthy social relationships, which are very much needed in the life of a person in recovery.

Determining which Program is Right for Your Loved One

Herein is the most challenging question parents and families face after it is determined that their loved one has an addiction, namely, determining which program is *right* for the addict? To assist in this matter, we will provide you with some principles to evaluate your circumstances. These are some fundamental questions a qualified inpatient admission director would ask. There are no black and white answers to this difficult question. Furthermore, *there is simply no replacement for getting a professional assessment.* What is offered below is not meant to supplant such an assessment. Each chemically-dependent person must be evaluated in order to "tailor make" a treatment program geared toward their needs.

The first inquiry that must be made should determine the primary drug of choice. The "drug of choice" (hereafter DOC) is the substance of which the chemically addicted person uses *most prevalently*. For instance, if a person uses alcohol, smokes marijuana, and heroin. Most likely, heroin is the "drug of choice" on the basis that if the addict had a choice they would probably choose heroin, since without it the addict would experience withdrawal. However, this is not a given. Typically, if the DOC is one of the "harder" drugs such as cocaine, heroin, methamphetamines more often than not inpatient treatment is necessary. However, DOC alone is not enough information to judge because at times marijuana users necessitate inpatient. What is more, in the case of alcoholism withdrawal, in some cases, is life threatening. This fact illustrates why professional guidance in the matter is vital. The DOC, therefore, influences what treatment is necessary. Another problem, which arises often, is that the parents or family know "something" is wrong but they're not sure exactly what chemical(s) the addict is using. In this case, it is helpful to have an idea what the general symptoms and behaviors of people under the influence of specific substances look like. If you are unable to discern what chemicals they are using or what their drug of choice is, that's okay. Move on to the next question.

Secondly, you need to determine if possible the "pattern" or "history" of their use. For instance, ever since Fred got injured in that car accident, he has been taking pain pills. That was over three years ago. It is helpful to try and establish how frequently the person uses. Knowing the frequency of their use will help you to determine the extent of treatment needed. If the person in question uses daily, it is much more likely he or she will need an inpatient or outpatient program simply because they offer more accountability. Experience has shown that those who use every day are more likely not to be able to control their impulses in a less-intensively sober environment. On the other hand, in the case of a high school student who gets pulled over with marijuana in the car. If he were not a daily or weekly user, it would be a little extreme to place him into an inpatient program. So each individual's *using pattern and behavior* will be a strong indicator of the level of rehabilitation necessary. Thus, someone who uses very frequently necessitates a more *intensive* treatment.

Also, attempt to find out the quantity (if possible) of chemicals the individual is consuming. This could be difficult in some situations, whereas it would be quite easy in others. In the case of an alcoholic it's generally easy to determine on average the daily consumption. Simply count the bottles or add up the amount of liquid consumed, unless the addict *hides the bottles*. Other chemicals like acid, ecstasy, heroin, cocaine, crack, and meth are more difficult because evidence usually isn't left out in the open. Quantity is also a significant indicator of placement into the different types of treatment. Alcoholism gives us a perfect example. A person who is consuming a liter of liquor a day will initially *have* to be put into an inpatient program. Since withdrawal from alcohol, if not medically supervised, can result in death, the individual's needs demand a medical inpatient detoxification. After the person has been medically cleared from the detoxification (removal of the presence of a chemical from body), then they can be assessed to determine further treatment options. From this example it is easy to see how the quantity of use can be such a vital indicator of the kind of rehab necessary.

Another major concern would be if your loved one has a psychiatric disorder. In the case of the addict having Bi-Polar disorder or Schizophrenia, they would require that these areas be addressed as well. Some treatment programs offer specialized care for this, which is commonly referred to as "dual-diagnoses" chemical dependency treatment. This means the patient is dealing with alcoholism/addiction and a psychiatric/mood disorder. If this is the case, other questions arise such as visits with psychiatrists, medication assessments, medication stabilization, etc. Also, some programs do not permit clients who take medication, these are usually the purely religious programs, nevertheless if the addict has a dual-diagnosis, in our opinion, *it is not advisable to place them in a program without properly trained medical professionals and access to proper medications.*

Thirdly, we want to concentrate on how erratic and dangerous the person's behavior is. Each unique human being has a different temperament under the influence of chemicals. Some are very predictable and calm while others are violent and unstable. In the case of a youth who is extremely defiant and leaves for extended periods of time, it would be advisable to place the individual in a "lock-up" or inpatient type of treatment center where he or she couldn't just run away because they didn't want to be there. Yet we still want to be sensitive to the middle-aged alcoholic who may drink a fifth of whiskey a day, but is not a violent or volatile personality. He may require intensive inpatient recovery treatment. However, he probably does *not* need to be in a "boot camp" type of program. Therefore, each circumstance should be individually assessed.

For our present consideration, the final major factor in determining the extent of treatment should be regarding the addict's legal complications. Chemically-dependent people normally travel with baggage. It is not without precedent for most addicts to bear the burden of significant legal problems, which sometimes are the stimuli driving them to treatment. Therefore, those legal matters that are outstanding should influence, to a degree, the type of treatment required. Also, they serve as a secondary indicator of the severity of the addictive problem. It is not uncommon for people to avoid the treatment they need until the court mandates them. There are forms of court mandated treatment that are within the walls of a prison also. Don't let the terminology confuse you, anything within the walls of a prison—is prison. One's legal issues and the severity of such should have an influence on the treatment they get. It is also true that legal problems are a peripheral issue in relation to treating the addiction. Nonetheless, it can be incredibly beneficial to attend an inpatient program, which tends to find favor with the court system. Frequently, judges are more favorable to an individual who has taken initiative to get help before the law mandates it.

There are many other questions that could be discussed. Unfortunately, we cannot cover them all, but what has been set forth above should outline the key factors in determining the appropriate solution for your loved one. Now let's explore some practical wisdom in light of finding the necessary help.

Peer Into My Life

I have personally attended different treatment programs in excess of nine times. Some of the treatment centers I have been admitted to were considered the *best* North America had to offer while others were not so famous. Here you will find my personal experience both as patient and administrator in the treatment industry.

Individual Counseling—My addiction was a little more extreme than most. During adolescence, my family sent me to numerous individual counselors. At this stage of my life, I was extremely defiant which detracted from this being exceptionally effectual, at least in my case. Granted I grew in many ways and undoubtedly was helped from my time in counseling, as far as addiction was concerned it did little if any good. What did occur was the beginnings of developing healthy communication skills and trust at a time when I trusted no one. Also, I think it's important for everyone to have people they can confide in and "bounce" ideas off of, which counseling did effectively.

Another downside, in my case, was that I was dishonest and a crafty manipulator. I used the counselor as leverage against my parents to get my way. For instance, I would present the "facts" from my perspective in a biased way, gaining the support of the counselor. Then in family sessions, I would use this to my advantage in manipulating my parents to allow me to do things they wouldn't normally do. I did this on the basis of justifying smoking cigarettes at a young age. After much work the counselor told my mom that in the scheme of things, she should probably let me smoke cigarettes. He told her to "choose her battles." I was twelve then and established through that a greater confidence in my own ability to manipulate. Therefore, if that can be done in my case, beware that the addict in your life might be just as capable to do the same.

A.A./N.A.—As a high school student, my addiction had progressed a great deal more than anyone else my age. I was drinking liquor and beer habitually both before and after school on a daily basis. In an attempt to save my life, my parents required daily attendance of A.A. meetings. So being the defiant addict that I was, I would drink before and after each meeting. Even though I didn't really work the program at that point, mere exposure to the lifestyle of recovery, the program of A.A./N.A., and the twelve steps helped me later in life. At the time when my addiction really started to wear on me, I was aware that there was help out there and knew where to go. The early exposure to A.A. in my life was instrumental in developing my character and self-awareness of addiction. I would never have been able to be effective working at a treatment center without my years of growing up in and around A.A..

As with most programs, A.A./N.A. won't produce fruit unless you put forth effort. Nobody can make your loved one stay clean. Yes, you can lock them up for a little while, but in the long run the desire to become sober has to come from inside them. For this reason, A.A. or N.A. is only helpful after someone has made a decision to quit using. Often inpatient treatment is necessary first.

Outpatient Treatment—I attended a few outpatient programs ranging from night classes to day-treatment programs. They substantially increased my understanding of addiction and the addictive process. Yet they were impotent in their ability to assist me in stopping the use of chemicals. This is because my addiction had progressed to the point that I didn't have the ability, even on a restricted schedule, to stop using. For me, if I wasn't in a controlled environment there was little doubt I would find some way to use chemicals. Of course, not everyone is in that position. I found that outpatient programs provided me with too much freedom for the severity of my case.

Inpatient Treatment—It was through inpatient treatment that God changed my life. Yet I went to many inpatient programs, prior to me actually putting together any extended period of sobriety. These programs provided a "controlled environment" that made a significant difference in my overall recovery. However, sometimes, as you should be cautioned ahead of time, illicit drugs find ways into inpatient programs. That simply goes with the territory and I am not familiar with a program anywhere in the country which has not struggled with that problem.

Generally, all inpatient programs offer educational classes. These classes cover an enormous plethora of recovery information ranging from "How did I get here?" to "Relapse Prevention." Education is essential to long term recovery in that if one doesn't understand why they use, they're destined to use again. Also, most inpatient programs offer individual counseling and/or therapy. This also is extremely helpful in sorting through the feelings and emotions a person goes through. Moreover, most addicts, as a result of their addiction, suffer from a lack of sufficient emotional development. That is, in relation to living on a day to day basis, addicts develop fragmented methods of coping with various emotional aspects of life, which must, in some sense, be rectified in order to recover. For instance, in my case, I started using drugs at a very early age. I taught myself to use chemicals in response to anger, loneliness, depression, etc. These behavioral responses to emotion had to be re-trained. Inpatient care helped me learn how to feel without using. This was facilitated through an environment with other recovering persons.

These programs provide the recovering person with a social environment. This environment provides a peer-group who are working through the same difficult issues. This fosters interpersonal relationships, bonds, and trust that have otherwise been damaged by addiction. Other programs do this as well, but not as efficiently as inpatient programs. Finally, inpatient programs allocate all of the patient's time and energy. Addicted persons tend to enjoy taking the "focus" off of them. So many people in outpatient or other programs focus on work, spouse, children, or hobbies rather than addressing the problem. Inpatient programs get the attention of those that are in them. This is very important. It is far too easy to become inundated with things other than addiction, leaving the sickness festering.

How Do I Find the Right Inpatient Program?

Finding the right program can mean the difference between life and death for the chemically-dependent person. Families who jump at the first program in the phonebook many times wind up having limited success, if any. Different programs offer different core fundamentals and can vary greatly. So families must know what the essentials are in selecting the correct program.

The essentials questions in finding the right inpatient program are:

1. *Tenure of Program*—Any reasonable person would be careful in selecting a surgeon for their sick child. This same caution should be used in finding a treatment program. There are many programs available. The question is not how they look, but their history and how they operate. A program's tenure (history) is important. You want to select a program that is not "fly-by-night." How long have they been helping people? Who administrates the program? Does anyone of reputable character recommend them?

2. *Core Beliefs*—What does the program teach? Do they teach the twelve-steps of A.A./N.A.? I think it is cause for alarm if they do not incorporate the twelve-steps somewhere in their program. Some programs operate with an exclusively spiritual approach which does work for some, but not everyone. What I call, a "balanced" program, which are few and far between, will offer both twelve-step and spiritual aspects. Be on guard also for programs with unorthodox core-beliefs. It has been my experience in the field that these programs do exist and can be dangerous. Always be upfront and ask what they believe and what they teach. Don't be afraid to ask to talk with some of their clients. Some top treatment programs won't allow you to do this based on "confidentiality," but it is still important to try and see how patients/clients view the program they're in. If you do talk to some clients, don't be surprised if they don't want to be there, because most people don't. The question that matters is whether the program is helping, not whether they "like" being there.

3. *Family Program*—One of the most overlooked areas in recovery is the family. Even though the family members may not be the ones with the addiction, they must be educated about both addiction and recovery as well. Indeed, the family must make changes too. This is usually resisted,

but the question is: how badly do you want you loved one to get better? Bad enough to change your lifestyle, too? The program you choose should have a family education program, family-support group, and should emphasize the importance of family involvement with the client.

4. *Length of Program*—The longer the program, the better—especially regarding inpatient programs. The more clean time the patients get, the better odds they have of staying clean for the duration. Thirty-day programs are common, but many times ineffective. This is because it takes about thirty days for an active user to regain a clear perception of reality. Never underestimate the importance of time in relation to successful sobriety.

5. *Spirituality*—Addiction is a spiritual problem as well as physical, mental, and emotional. To leave the spiritual part un-addressed is to make an all-too-common fatal mistake. Many programs boast spirituality, yet in reality their "spirituality" is more man-centered than God-centered. I encourage you to sincerely attempt to find a Christian program. They have a higher success rate in general than secular treatments. The difficulty is usually in finding a Christian program that incorporates the 12-Steps and group therapy also.

6. *Individual/Group Counseling/Therapy*—It is important that your loved one get the help they need. You want to find a program with a balanced counseling agenda. Group therapy is vital and should be a larger part of the program than individual. Yet individual therapy is important in the process as well. Be wary of any program that only uses one rather than both models of individual and group counseling/therapy.

7. *Client/Patient responsibility*—By responsibilities here we mean chores or some type of work-like activity. Some programs, especially the so-called "insurance giants," have few if any client/patient responsibilities. This means in the end that your loved one isn't being required to become independent and self-maintaining. Programs that have few patient responsibilities foster recovering persons who remain more dependent in the long run. The benefit of client/patient responsibility is that it brings about stronger character and more self-confidence, not to mention more adult-like maturity.

8. *Activities*—Any good program will offer activities to their patients. Unless your loved one is an "out-of-control" adolescent, stay away

from treatment programs that keep their patients locked-up inside of a building. Don't misunderstand, most inpatient programs are locked up to some degree. You want to find one that, as much as possible, provides your loved one with relative freedom. The less they feel trapped, the better they will respond.

Half-Way Houses and Recovery Homes

Halfway houses (otherwise known as recovery homes) are generally post-treatment opportunities, though not always. They are homes within a city or town in which 3–8 recovering persons live. They generally work during the day and are required by the house to attend a certain number of meetings and/or church services. They provide their residents with ample opportunity to get plugged back into society while still having some accountability.

Usually, it is inappropriate to place someone in a recovery home who hasn't had at least thirty or more days clean and sober. As stated previously, recovery homes are best for those who have just completed a treatment program. This phase of recovery allows them to be integrated back into the workforce, begin attending meetings (being personally responsible), and actually staying clean and sober in the real world. Since there is a great deal of added freedom in the recovery home setting, it is unwise for someone with little or no clean time to live at one. They will most likely continue using and could adversely affect the recovery of those living in the home.

There Is Help

There is help for you and your family. No matter how bad your present circumstance may be, *there is help.* Even the most tragic addiction can be turned around. A director of one of the top programs in the nation told my mother there wasn't help for someone like me. She couldn't even give us a referral to a program that offered the kind of "extensive" help she was sure I needed. Indeed, in her opinion, I was headed for prison with little hope of recovery. Isiah Robertson, the founder/director of House of Isaiah, a long-term recovery center for men, didn't feel the same way. He saw my checkered past and treatment history as a challenge, which God and treatment could change. He was right. Today, I am pursuing my life's dreams, working on graduate education, I'm married to the woman of my dreams and have a family. Indeed, my relationship with my own parents has been

12

What Will a Good Program Teach?

Assuming that you have found or are evaluating a program that you believe is right for your loved one. What should you expect them to learn in treatment? What will a good program give them? What coping skills and recovery tools are necessary to help them stay clean? As has been established previously, a quality chemical-dependency treatment program should be able to provide your loved one with a safe chemical-free environment. The atmosphere should be one that promotes recovery and emphasizes life without using chemicals. It should emphasize rehabilitation of the "whole" man, which is comprised of spirit/soul/mind and body. Rehabilitation is a compilation of education, life skills, emotional growth, and practical application. These four categories are essential to any successful rehabilitation program. We will define further each category, emphasizing those key elements, which make a rehabilitation program impact the lives of its patients.

Education

We find that human behavior is an expression of our "inner realities." Here we want to focus on the information we take in, in relation to the formation of the "inner realities." Thus, the information we take in directly affects our perception of the world and therefore, the way in which we relate to the world. Or to express it differently Matthew records Jesus expressing the point in this way: "For where your treasure is, there will your heart be also. The light of the body is the eye: if therefore thine eye be single, thy whole body shall be full of light." (Matt. 6:21–22 NKJV). This passage indicates that the eye is a "gate," in some sense, to the soul. Whatever the eye is focused on penetrates the heart. This applies with any of our audio/visual senses. What we listen to gets into our minds. What we watch on television affects our thinking.

This truth puts the importance and relevance of education at an even higher premium. Therefore, recovery education is the foundation for change. To change an addict's behavior, they must be educated about the problem and the solution. Addressing both issues is paramount. First, a quality program will emphasize education about addiction from the perspective of the problem. This should start with the topic of why the chemically dependent person is in rehabilitation. Hopefully, this will provide needed answers to the client about why treatment is necessary and what they can hope to accomplish with the opportunity to be in rehabilitation.

Further education about the problem would include information about the disease concept of addiction. Teaching the client what their problem is in an understandable way, which they can relate to, is foundational to long-term recovery. If the addict does not understand the elementary principles of addiction, how can they be expected to sustain long-term sobriety? For this reason, proper education in addiction is vital. Each client should be presented with enough high-quality chemical dependency information to grasp the addictive process. This grasp will assist them in the future in staying sober. Along with understanding addiction, other characteristics must be addressed educationally.

Clients need adequate instruction regarding the emotions which foster addiction. Some of the most important topics are denial, rationalization, feelings, loneliness, and coping skills. Part of the power to overcome these obstacles is in understanding them. Many times, the chemically dependent person isn't even aware of their participation in these behaviors. Accompanying education about the problem should be concrete lessons that provide the client with viable solutions. Simply understanding the problem won't help anyone stay sober. That is why it is so imperative that a treatment program educate your loved one extensively on the solution. Many times this means learning the twelve-steps of Alcoholics Anonymous/Narcotics Anonymous. The twelve steps are a pattern laid out in "steps" which can potentially provide a new way of life. They have been and continue to be instrumental in the sobriety of literally millions around the world.

What Do the Twelve Steps Teach?

Each step focuses on a vital concept to sustaining daily sobriety from alcohol and other chemicals. For instance the first step reads, "We came to believe that we were powerless over alcohol and our lives became unmanageable."[1] Keep in mind in any of the A.A. steps a drug addict would

---

1. The steps listed below are from *Alcoholics Anonymous* [4th edition], 59–60. The following articulation of the twelve-steps is not A.A. approved, that is, the views expressed here

simply exchange the word "alcohol" for heroin, cocaine, or whatever their drug of choice may be. The first step addresses the problem. Until one comes to grips with their own inability to stop using of their own accord, they can't begin to recover. One fatal characteristic of addiction is the unique defense of one's own inability. For some reason, one of the hardest things to get a chemically-dependent person to do is to recognize they can't stop on their own.

On its face, this doesn't seem as though it should be so great a road-block, but it is. Virtually every addict hates to admit utter defeat. Recovery is the one distinct realm in which the only way to win is to surrender! This paradox, I think, has baffled addicted persons for a long time. Yet a program of recovery prescribes first and foremost recognition of powerlessness and unmanageability. Unless a person's life is unmanageable and they lack sufficient power to remedy the situation, why would they need help at all? The second step says, "Came to believe that a power greater than ourselves could restore us to sanity." This is the ultimate purpose of recovery: restoration. Yet this A.A. step slaps the humanistic "I can do it myself" personality right in the face. To go any further in recovery, one must pursue a power outside of themselves. While A.A. here leaves it explicitly open to interpretation, it is my experience that only the Christian God is sufficient for this role, though my opinion in the field is not without its critics. What is exceptionally beneficial is that A.A. makes the need for a spiritual solution evident. Restoration requires a spiritual solution as well as emotive and cognitive solutions. Interestingly, there is an element both of surrender in this step as well as insufficiency, when one asserts their own insanity regarding addiction/alcoholism.

What constitutes insanity is the addiction itself, doing the same thing over and over, while expecting different consequences. Each day the addict puts chemicals into their body. Each time they have a horrible reaction and their lives tragically get worse. Yet day after day, they do the same action, expecting this time to be different. That is insanity. Step three says, "Made a decision to turn our will and our life over to the care of God as we understand him." This step develops the previous step by taking it to the next level. Therefore, it is clear that the steps are meant to follow a logical order.

Now the addict/alcoholic must make a decision. This decision is one of significant importance. Indeed, it is to turn over their will and life to God. So in order to complete step three, one must have come to an understanding of God as part of completing step two. The concept

are the author's *interpretation* of the benefit and meaning of the twelve-steps.

of recovering persons having a spiritual life again is emphasized strongly. Steps one through three thus far have called the prospective recoveree to some serious realizations. First, powerlessness and unmanageability were addressed giving the addict/alcoholic sufficient *need* to work a recovery program. Secondly, it established a consciousness of and necessity for a relationship with God. Then it joins both concepts by placing dependence upon God as the source of restoration.

Next, step four, "Made a searching and fearless moral inventory of ourselves." The program's focus now takes an introspective turn. This challenges the recovering person to take "inventory." An inventory is a detailed appraisal that reports all materials and goods within a certain range. In this context, the "range" would be the recovering person's life. This would include family, friends, and any other interpersonal relationships. A moral inventory would be an assessment of moral values. A.A. seems highly interested in bringing to light the underlying values systems which determine behavior, a point we stressed earlier.

Once the personal inventory has been accomplished, then it is time to take action with these findings. Step five says, "Admitted to God, to ourselves, and to another human being the exact nature of our wrongs." Here there are a number of interesting requirements for the addict/alcoholic. Again we find that step five cannot be accomplished without previously completing step four. Indeed, step five requires communication. By this step, the addicted person is asked to face "the exact nature of our wrongs." That equates to an honest evaluation of past behavior and present attitudes. This is a crucial turning point in the progression of the steps. It is here that the chemically-addicted person can ultimately be rigorously honest or not. If the latter occurs the addict, in all probability, will simply return to or continue in the addicted self-deception. However, if the former occurs this honest turn would mean breaking free from the yoke of secrecy.

Two of the most powerful barriers to sobriety for the addict are secrecy and shame. They go hand in hand since shame fosters secrecy. The more secrecy, the more deception. Deception keeps the addict sick. So this step helps break the tireless cycle of destruction. In completing this step, one could undergo a miraculous change. I have known many alcoholics who consider this step the turning point in their recovery. That is not to say the other steps couldn't produce the same effect for different people. It should be further noted here that step five should be done with a sponsor/mentor. This information should not be shared abroad. It is not necessary for the addict to confess their transgressions to everyone over and over. This step is about building trust, getting honest, and addressing issues head on. Be careful to realize the sensitive nature of this information. This should not be shared with a parent, family member, or simply a friend.

Step six is, "Were entirely ready to have God remove these defects of character." Real recovery is about change. Change occurs from the inside out. The relation and progression of the steps should be more obvious now, as six flows naturally out of five. When working step five, the addict shared their exhaustive moral inventory. This brought to light their "character defects." These are the things in their character, what all people have to some extent, that have been found to be liabilities rather than assets. This step allows the recovering person the opportunity to realize, evaluate, and render powerless these "liabilities" in their character. Since these character defects are flaws within one's own character, the removal requires power outside of oneself, namely, God's help. Notice how successfully working the A.A. program involves a humble request of grace from God. It is only God who has the power of deliverance. He is the only one who can "deliver" your loved one from themselves.

Step seven, "Humbly ask Him to remove our shortcomings." This step is the action following step six. Each step builds upon the work of the prior step. Since step seven is primarily an action-completing step, little needs to be said here concerning it. The eighth step of Alcoholics Anonymous is, "Made a list of all persons we had harmed and became willing to make amends to them all." This is terrifying to most addicts. Addiction cultivates destruction and this step causes the addict to compile a list of people they have directly hurt emotionally, physically or both during their active using.

Making an amend means admitting guilt and attempting to repair an offense between two individuals. This step requires the individual not only to accumulate a list of amends that need to be made, but also calls for the willingness to make the amends. One has not thoroughly completed an "eighth" step until they have become willing to make the amends. Next is step nine, "Made direct amends to such people except when to do so would injure themselves or others." This is a scary proposition regardless of whether you are an addict or not. Making amends to people we have harmed is very humbling. Yet that is the ninth step to recovery in A.A.'s opinion.

One of the most powerful victories in recovery is finding out that life goes on after making amends. The ninth step is all about overcoming obstacles that seem impenetrable. The victory comes when you face people you didn't think you could and when you put to rest things, situations, and people that you've been using chemicals *at* for years. Steps five through nine are chiefly concerned with action. They are the "works" of recovery that must be done to clean house. I think each of these steps are well founded in biblical-principles and should not cause any concern for the Christian; in fact, it would seem that these fundamentally embody the essence of Christian reconciliation.

The final three steps are termed by many as "maintenance" steps. The reason for this is because each step ensures the continuity of healthy recovery. They keep the recovering person continually growing closer to God and being quick to see their own faults in situations.

Step ten says, "Continued to take personal inventory and when we were wrong promptly admitted it." As if making the first fearless and moral inventory weren't enough, step ten provides the opportunity to never have to make such a difficult moral inventory again by taking a daily inventory. This prevents one from storing up "skeletons" that must be dealt with later. It also provides a provision for continual introspection. This promotes the longevity of recovery by requiring the individual to always look inward. At the same time, it keeps one open to seeing "their part" of given situations. If every person would work the tenth step everyday, this world would be a much different place. The eleventh step says, "We sought through prayer and meditation to improve our conscious contact with God as we understand him. Praying only for the knowledge of his will for us and the power to carry that out." The emergence of a spiritual life comes to a head in step eleven. Now the addict/alcoholic agrees to seek a more deep interpersonal relationship with God.

This step even goes as far as to say that the recovering person would spend time seeking the will of God for his or her life and the power to carry that out. Step eleven really makes it difficult for any person who chooses a rock or the ceiling fan as their higher power. Now the nuts and bolts of spirituality are to come to the knowledge of God's will and the willingness and submission to live in accordance with it. Concluding our myriad of recovery, we top our recovery tree with a beautiful ornament: step twelve. "Having had a spiritual awakening as a result of these steps, we tried to carry this message to alcoholics and to practice these principles in all our affairs." This step reveals clearly the intent of the "steps," namely, to bring about psychic change.

Notice the directive to serve other people, post-spiritual awakening. What a marvelous concept. After getting clean, working the steps, and having a spiritual awakening, now take what you've received and help someone else. There is a saying in the rooms of A.A. that goes like this, "You've got to give it away, to keep it." This means if you don't help others, you'll never fully realize your own recovery. True recovery embodies helping others to attain what once seemed so impossible for you. It is our hope that you now have a brief understanding of what the twelve steps of A.A. consist of and a relative apprehension of why. These steps should be taught to your loved one in hopes that they follow these steps and reap the bountiful spiritual fruit millions have found in them. Never allow your church group to slander the A.A. program based on their own ignorance of the program.

Spiritual Education

We have clearly established that chemical dependency is a spiritual problem. So any education hoping to aid addicted persons would be deficient if it lacked spirituality. This topic, as with politics, is most controversial. There are many different views of what constitutes spirituality. We have here taken an expressly Christian viewpoint. Not everyone reading this will agree, however, the author's perspective will frame what is below.

Due to the variety of Christian sects and other religious expressions in our society, it is necessary for recovering persons who are expected to develop a relationship with God to know something about him. This is where spiritual education comes in. "How are they to call on one they have not believed in? And how are they to believe in one they have not heard of? And how are they to hear without someone preaching to them?" (Romans 10:14, NET) Paul words this paradox marvelously. People must be taught about God. For how will they grow without a teacher? Recovering persons must be educated in what the Scriptures teach. The Word of God is the source of truth. The closer the recovering person becomes acquainted with the Scripture, the better equipped they are to live in righteousness.

There is no denomination which has a corner on the market of recovery or deliverance. So in no way do we promote a specific denomination. We promote a personal relationship with Jesus Christ. Few treatment programs will offer Jesus *and* also the twelve steps. This is a travesty. Successful programs effectively communicate *both* the Word of God and the recovery program of A.A./N.A.. A proper spiritual education program will provide for all the essentials. These are the fundamentals of the Christian faith. This is so each person has a firm understanding of salvation, water baptism, the person of the Holy Spirit, basic bible study, prayer, and worship. These elements will equip them to sustain and nourish their relationship with God through His Son, Jesus Christ.

It is highly recommended that the program you select have a daily Bible study or spiritual curriculum. The reason for this, as with A.A./N.A., is to provide your loved one with consistency, which with the help of God can become a habit. The great hope of treatment is that the habits developed in treatment will supplant the habits of using. Below are some foundational Scriptures I encourage you to memorize. Do it slowly by memorizing one or two a week. These will prove essential to you in your own recovery. Suggest them also to your loved one. You can even require it if you have to. These Scriptures changed my life. They will change yours, too, if you will give them a chance.

(All Scripture references from the *English Standard Version.*)

> Call to me and I will answer you, and will tell you great and hidden things that you have not known. (Jeremiah 33:3)

> Do not be anxious about anything, but in everything by prayer and supplication with thanksgiving let your requests be made known to God. (Philippians 4:6)

> My people are destroyed for lack of knowledge; because you have rejected knowledge, I reject you from being a priest to me. And since you have forgotten the law of your God, I also will forget your children. (Hosea 4:6)

> No temptation has overtaken you that is not common to man. God is faithful, and he will not let you be tempted beyond your ability, but with the temptation he will also provide the way of escape that you may be able to endure it. (1 Corinthians 10:13)

> For the weapons of our warfare are not of the flesh but have divine power to destroy strongholds. We destroy arguments and every lofty opinion raised against the knowledge of God, and take every thought captive to obey Christ. (2 Corinthians 10:4–5)

> Not that I have already obtained this or am already perfect, but I press on to make it my own, because Christ Jesus has made me his own. Brothers, I do not consider that I have made it my own. But one thing I do: forgetting what lies behind and straining forward to what lies ahead, I press toward the goal for the prize of the upward call of God in Christ Jesus. (Philippians 3:12–14)

Finally, all of you, have unity of mind, sympathy, brotherly love, a tender heart and a humble mind. Do not repay evil for evil or reviling for reviling, but on the contrary, bless, for to this you were called, that you may obtain a blessing. (1 Peter 3:8–9)

Beloved, do not be surprised at the fiery trial when it comes upon you to test you, as though something strange were happening to you. But rejoice insofar as you share Christ's sufferings, that you may also rejoice and be glad when his glory is revealed. (1 Peter 4:12–13)

And we know that for those who love God all things work together for good, for those who are called according to his purpose. (Romans 8:28)

If we say we have no sin, we deceive ourselves, and the truth is not in us. If we confess our sins, he is faithful and just to forgive us our sins and to cleanse us from all unrighteousness. If we say we have not sinned, we make him a liar, and his word is not in us. (1 John 1:8–10)

Toward the scorners he is scornful, but to the humble he gives favor. The wise will inherit honor, but fools get disgrace. (Proverbs 3:34–35)

But they who wait for the Lord shall renew their strength; they shall mount up with wings like eagles; they shall run and not be weary; they shall walk and not faint. (Isaiah 40:31)

I can do all things through him who strengthens me. (Philippians 4:13)

Count it all joy, my brothers, when you meet trials of various kinds, for you know that the testing of your faith produces steadfastness. And let steadfastness have its full effect, that you may be perfect and complete, lacking in nothing. (James 1:2–4)

Now faith is the assurance of things hoped for, the conviction of things not seen. (Hebrews 11:1)

If God is for us, who can be against us? (Romans 8:31)

So Jesus said to the Jews who had believed in him, "If you abide in my word, you are truly my disciples, and you will know the truth, and the truth will set you free; So if the Son sets you free, you will be free indeed." (John 8:31–32,36)

Moses said to the people, "Do not fear, for God has come to test you, that the fear of him may be before you, that you may not sin." (Exodus 20:20)

Whoever finds his life will lose it, and whoever loses his life for my sake will find it. (Matthew 10:39)

Come to me, all who labor and are heavy laden, and I will give you rest. (Matthew 11:28)

Blessed is the man who remains steadfast under trial, for when he has stood the test he will receive the crown of life, which God has promised to those who love him. (James 1:12)

For you know that afterward, when he desired to inherit the blessing, he was rejected, for he found no chance to repent, though he sought it with tears. (Hebrews 12:17)

For I am sure that neither death nor life, nor angels nor rulers, nor things present nor things to come, nor powers, nor height nor depth, nor anything else in all creation, will be able to separate us from the love of God in Christ Jesus our Lord. (Romans 8:38–39)

Do you not know that in a race all the runners compete, but only one receives the prize? So run that you may obtain it. Every athlete exercise self-control in all things. They do it to receive a perishable wreath, but we an imperishable. So I do not run aimlessly; I do not box as one beating the air. But I discipline my body and keep it under control, lest after preaching to others I myself should be disqualified. (1 Corinthians 9:24–27)

What If My Loved One Doesn't Believe in God?

Many families of chemically addicted persons struggle with the question, "What if my loved one doesn't believe in God?" First, you need to know that this is not uncommon. Beliefs can change. Don't allow their present "disbelief" to discourage you. Not all Christian programs have a prerequisite of being a Christian before you come to the program. For instance, let's take a few moments and allow me to share with you some experience from my own life. During the course of my life, my mother attempted to lead me back into relationship with God as I had previously had in my early childhood. She tried many times to tell me about God when I was struggling in life.

Each time, I dismissed her ideas and her God. I wanted nothing to do with "God," for a number of reasons I had devised. My reasoning was that "religion" was simply a crutch for weak people who needed to believe in something to help them get through life. I had a plethora of disputes to each of her attempts to get me right with God. Yet even as adamant and stubborn as I had been, God still chose to breath life into my soul and illuminate me to the person and work of Jesus Christ. It really didn't happen until I had been in a Christian program for a few months. It didn't happen the first day or the first month, for that matter. I didn't want to go to Bible study every morning (It was part of the program.). It was in those Bible studies that I didn't want to attend and I tried not to pay attention that God showed up in my life. Never allow your loved one's present spiritual disposition or lack thereof to sway your choosing a Christian program. All the excuses in the world couldn't convince me not to send my own child to a Christian program. The reality is that you, whether you're the parents, family, or spouse must make the right decision. When you let the addict prescribe their own treatment, you're already in trouble.

Recovery Education

The term recovery education is a general term which encompasses all the topics that are vital to recovery, yet don't fall under spirituality or the Twelve-steps. This educational information should cover topics such as how to live with yourself, feelings (from a different perspective than above), relationship communication, working your program, and relapse prevention. While these subjects may not find themselves under the distinguished categories like spirituality and the Twelve-steps they, nevertheless, are important. The subject of feelings is a broad topic, which we have mentioned numerous times.

Hopefully, the following will help you to have a more concrete idea of what we mean when we say feelings. If you question an addict as to why they used in a specific instance, they will usually respond with a feeling such as, "I was *lonely, tired, angry, etc.*" The reason is because addiction is a feeling driven disease. Addicts tend to be "feeling" junkies. Their emotions have supreme reign over their behavior. They use because they feel different emotions. Since no human is capable of ceasing to feel emotion, the addict must learn a new way to deal with their feelings effectively. Our purpose is to educate those in early recovery to modify their reactionary behavior when they feel specific emotions. So when they feel angry, tired, lonely etc., rather than using, they will call a sponsor, go to a meeting, or pray. Relationship communication is another skill that most chemically dependent persons lack. During the course of most addictions; the addict's interpersonal relationship skills become skewed. This results in an inability to communicate with family and friends competently. With the proper education, however, the addict can again become proficient in communicating in a healthy way.

As you can see recovery education is essential to the recovery process of any chemically-dependent person. Be sure that the treatment program you have selected emphasizes the many topics of recovery education. Ensuring that they do, could affect the long-term recovery of your loved one. When choosing a program, education should be a major thrust of the program. All three subjects (spirituality, recovery, and twelve-steps) should be taught to provide your loved one with the very best opportunity to recover. Many addicts maintian long-term recovery because of comprehensive education they received in treatment.

Life Skills

One of the most overlooked areas of recovery treatment is the subject of life skills. Life skills are the basic skills that are needed to sustain independent life in society. This may sound very simple but you would be amazed to find out how many addicted persons don't know how to make a resume or manage their checkbook. For many addicts, they missed some of the most elementary lessons of life while using. Shame sadly cloaks this deficiency, keeping the addict stuck in a state of inability both to manage the basic skills of life and also keep from asking for help. A quality recovery program will offer some kind of life skills education.

Emotional Growth

Any treatment should facilitate the opportunity for emotional growth. This should be not only on the individual level, but also corporately. Since many times it is essential for the addicted person and close relatives (family/spouse) to be separate during the treatment process, it is vital that there be a "therapeutic community." A therapeutic community is a clinical word to describe a group living situation of recovering persons. This environment stimulates emotional and psychological growth. It will be in these communities that your loved one will learn how to live with others successfully. It will also provide ample opportunities for your loved one to grow. Growth is stimulated by discomfort. Usually people don't change when things are comfortable. It won't hurt your loved one long-term for them to experience some discomfort in treatment. In fact, it might benefit them exceedingly. So a quality program will provide a group community that fosters interpersonal relationships with others in recovery.

It is imperative that as the family, you understand that your loved one's "comfort" is not paramount. We are not in any way insinuating that your loved one should experience un*suitable* living situations. What we are saying is that just because your loved one doesn't like their roommate, or the room they're in, or the fact that they have been moved a few times to different beds around the facility is not reason for you to become upset or involved.

Practical Application

Practical application is where the rubber meets the road, that is, the intersection of theory and practice. Any effective treatment program should offer many versatile activities to encourage the application or practice of those things taught in the classroom. Without question, I believe practical application to be the central focus of inpatient treatment. It is one thing to have a cerebral knowledge of recovery, yet it is something much different to practice what you preach! *When the addict learns by experience in a treatment community, the quality of that experience is priceless.* What can a program offer to cultivate practical application experiences? Effectual treatment programs should offer three primary activities to assist their clients in practically applying what they have been taught. These three are: communal living environments, physical activities, and client responsibilities/government.

None of the above listed three will be laid out for you in any treatment brochure. These are things you must actively look for to ensure that your client is receiving at the program you have selected for them. Communal living environments provide ample opportunity for interaction between clients. This gives them the opportunity to empathize with others' difficulties. Also, they can begin to communicate their own emotions and struggles. The sharing of these intimate details will create bonds between the clients which can be very beneficial to their long-term recovery.

Physical activities offer much more than their physical benefit alone. Sports and other activities develop skills in how to be part of a team. They deepen trust between clients and foster the "team" mentality. It is important for your loved one to find comradery in the recovering lifestyle. Loners in recovery are like lone sheep; they get devoured by the wolves. Physical activities should come in a variety of outlets providing clients the opportunity to find those activities they enjoy. Client responsibilities and government are vital to the recovery process of your loved one also. Treatment programs which facilitate client responsibilities, however, are rare. Nevertheless, a quality program will teach your loved one personal responsibility to the corporate body by giving them chores. These chores could be anything from shopping for groceries, cleaning, cooking, laundry, etc.

You want to ensure that the program you have chosen facilitates personal responsibility. There are programs available where the client's food is prepared, laundry is done for them, and other needs are taken care of in an effort to encourage a "focus on recovery." Don't be misled —these programs are generally not very beneficial even though they are "comfortable." Recovery involves responsibility. Excellent treatment programs will make possible sufficient opportunity to learn and practice responsibility.

Conclusion

Your understanding of what your loved one is learning in treatment is important. It's vital to their recovery and your own. The more you understand addiction and treatment the better equipped you will be to participate as a healthy influence in the life of your loved one. With a proper understanding, you, too, can *Recover All!*

13

What Is Relapse?

THE SUBJECT of relapse is one of great controversy within the field of chemical dependency. Out of all the various topics that fall under the umbrella of addiction, relapse happens to be the taboo. Its formal definition isn't hard to find, but for many it is a difficult situation to explain. Relapse occurs if and when the recovering person uses chemicals after being clean for any period of time. For instance, suppose Billy went to treatment for thirty days. He then came home to his parents' house and got a job. Three weeks later, he used. That is called relapse. However, conversely if Billy never actually got clean, he wouldn't be "relapsing," he would still be in active using.

Together we will explore a case of relapse in the life of an actual recovering person. When it comes to relapse, there are few, if any, concrete answers. Ultimately, it boils down to ingesting chemicals, but for the addict, it is much more than that. Relapse starts far before actual use takes place. To help illustrate this complex subject matter, we will look at my personal experience in the struggle to recover from crack cocaine.

Why Does Relapse Happen?

Relapse can't happen if there isn't some foundation of recovery to relapse from. What we mean here is that one actually has to *be clean* to relapse. You can't *re*-lapse until you have sobriety from which to lapse, if that makes sense. So in this section, we will look explicitly at one of the most tragic years of my addiction and recovery. What you will gain below is the addict's perspective of the events leading up to one of my many relapses along the road of getting clean.

At the age of 20, I was physically, emotionally, and every other way worn to the bone with my addiction. At this point, I had personally visited as a patient at least 8 different inpatient treatments. We had already exhausted individual drug and alcohol counseling and other similar programs. The dark clouds of using loomed, casting their shadows upon my soul. During the course of my addiction thus far, I had sold all my possessions more than once. I had broken in my own parents' home and stolen from them, even stooping to the all-time low of stealing family heirlooms for drug money.

When I drank alcohol, no longer was it for fun or excitement. The reality is that my drinking had gotten so bad, even I didn't like who it made me. Yet it was a compulsion, a necessity. I needed it. Considering my background, the kind of family I was from, and all the opportunities that were offered me, my life was genuinely a disgrace. What had looked like such a promising life, through my addiction, had been brought crumbling down. My memories were infested with misery that I had brought on through years of drug use. Indeed, I was demonized by my past, images that wouldn't leave my mind of places I had seen and terrible things I had done. In typical fashion, my family had convened after one of my recent alcoholic episodes in order to attempt to determine the right course of action for my life. They wanted to help me get on the right track. This time, the outlook was most grim. Everyone involved was at a loss for what to do with me. All the options had been exhausted. There were fewer and fewer ideas of what would help. Of course, I was no stranger to despair; so blindly, as a boy whistling in the dark, I told my family *this time I really can get clean, just give me the chance.* This, however, was not the first time they had heard this line from me.

We resolved that day to let me try it one more time. I would attend A.A. everyday—sometimes twice a day. After thirty days, I could find a job and begin to try and build a somewhat normal life. My family was just hoping I could live day to day without using drugs. That in itself would take a miracle. I determined within myself that at any cost I would give my best effort to staying clean and sober. I was so tired of my life being miserable. This, I thought, would be the opportunity to finally turn my misguided life around. It was now time to dig in and get serious. Whatever the cost, my resolve was to do it.

With this in mind, there were some other factors that were important in the landscape of my life at that time. Not only was the attempt at staying clean and sober a slow and painful start, but I had to learn how to live without the "love of my life," both of them, actually. Kristi, my long-time girlfriend, left me. She was my best friend (next to chemicals), who had lived with me for two years. It was the longest relationship I'd ever had at that point in my life. She was also my partner in crime. She loved drugs as much as I did, so in that regard we were "made" for each other. Indeed, we thought, quite immaturely, that we would be together forever, but that too was a pipe dream. When my addiction got so bad that I actually had to try and get clean and sober, she opted out. Her heart was with the drugs, not me. So after a fight, she moved out of my place and in with an old boyfriend. And just like that, she was gone.

For a long period of time, each day felt very dark and lonely. For an addict who didn't fare well when it came to dealing with emotions to begin with, it was a hard time. In reality, I probably never could have gotten clean around her, but at the time no one could have convinced me of that. This time, I would have to start over without her, in recovery. Relapse was the only consistent behavior I had ever known and now I felt alone and depressed, and especially hopeless. In an effort to soothe the pain, I went to church. It seemed to me that if there was a God, I probably needed Him as much as anybody did. My motives were selfish at first, looking for what I could get from Him, but who isn't, initially? Being the dramatic and overly-driven person that I am, I jumped into the church scene with both feet, so to speak. My personality, as is common with addicts, couldn't simply participate in an activity; my whole life had to be consumed with whatever the activity was.

On another front, the people in the Alcoholics Anonymous program embraced me with open arms. Even though I was young, they appreciated what I had to say and listened to me. Associating with so many adults didn't bother me either; in fact, I was probably more comfortable around adults. Thank God, the people at A.A. were understanding of my plight. The scariest place emotionally for me was to be alone. I loathed being alone. Some fear death, others fear disaster, my fear was being alone and those were the exact circumstances I found myself in. From my perspective, I was enduring some of the most difficult days emotionally of my life. So day after day, I "worked" the program and attended meetings. I even got a sponsor. (A sponsor is a type of mentor that, in principle, should assist the sponsee in working the steps.)

This time I was determined not to fail. So when I chose my sponsor, I picked him because he "had what I wanted." Little did I know he was really serious about working the steps. All things considered it turned out to be a great relationship; he demanded a great deal from me, which for me was very beneficial. Also, he happened to be involved in a small community of young people who were clean and sober. These young adults had "meetings" outside of meetings, that is, they would have A.A.-type meetings in their home. They also went out together socially. This was definitely a "God thing" for me, in that, I needed friendships with people my age.

It wasn't long before I put 60 days clean and sober together. I was going strong and it seemed as though nothing could move me. I got a job managing a cellular phone store and within a short time they promoted me and I was given a store of my own to manage. Everything, it seemed, was "turning to roses." My family was exceptionally pleased and I was happy, though there still seemed to be a "void" I needed to fill—I longed for a relationship. That was my weak link—I was desperate for a relationship with the opposite sex. Parenthetically, and in retrospect, this was resultant of issues I needed to deal with, and had little to do with a real "need" for a relationship, but even being cognizant of that fact probably wouldn't have deterred my determination to meet Mrs. Right. Indeed, I missed the attention, affection, and joy of being in a committed relationship. So, needless to say, I was constantly on the prowl.

One day, I had the ingenious idea to meet someone on one of the "matching" websites on the internet. Being a store manager enabled me to have "down time" at work and access to the internet. So I posted my profile and began searching. I even had a strategic plan, as was characteristic of my personality. I would simply email every single attractive woman and just like any mass-marketing program, wait for my two percent response. Well, my two percent response was little to be excited about. A few of the individuals I met were nice, but none of them were remotely what I was looking for. This process was very disappointing, since even though I was desperate, it wasn't a blind or thoughtless desperation. Therefore, the failure in meeting someone desirable forced me to, by default, spend time becoming more spiritual, that is, I attempted prayer and Bible study.

Then I got an unexpected response from a woman on the internet. She said she was an LSU student. She came from a very wealthy family in the New Orleans area. Her name was Amy. She seemed to be both beautiful and kind so needless to say, we hit it off immediately, at least on the phone. We talked for hours and hours each day and night. Soon I was planning how we were going to see each other. I guess the monotony got to her first, because before I knew it, she drove to Texas to see me. I was actually startled when I met her because she was so much more beautiful than any of the women I had met thus far online. There were indeed some strange things about her, but I didn't pay attention to the "little" details. I wanted to fall in love, and she was as good a candidate as any.

So before long, my imagination and common sense seemed to dissipate. My family was happy that I was happy, so there wasn't much they could say. Soon I began flying back and forth between Texas and New Orleans for visits. Before long, she began to share with me the "skeletons" in her closet. It turns out that Amy was a recovering anorexic. Her anorexia had at one time in her life become so advanced that she had to drop out of college. During that time, she had been hospitalized on numerous occasions and was presently in intensive therapy for the disorder. This was news to me, but because I was in recovery, I didn't think it would be an issue. If anything, maybe we could "help" each other since we were both in recovery.

At first, her disorder seemed like a workable challenge. So after we spent a few weeks together, being the patient recovering addict that I was, I purchased a ring and asked her to marry me. (Remember, I don't do anything halfway.) She accepted and the planning began. Everything was going wonderfully, it seemed. It was apparent from her behavior in intimate situations that something wasn't "normal." Then she told me about her history of sexual abuse. She explained to me graphically how her father, a powerful attorney in New Orleans, had sexually molested her on and off for over 15 years. I personally have never experienced sexual abuse. At best my understanding of the outworkings of abuse, were limited. In reality, I had no idea what I was involved with. Later, she would tell me that at various times she would hallucinate seeing her father's face on other people. I kept telling myself that surely she would feel safer and get over some of the hang-ups with time. I reasoned that if I could recover, so could she. So, rather than giving up, I decided to stick it out with her.

Then, one weekend while I stayed at her parents home in New Orleans her sister, Caroline, came home from the college she was attending in Florida. It was apparent the sisters weren't that close. There was much bad blood between them. I wasn't sure yet why, but there was something. Caroline drank alcoholically, something that became glaringly obvious only having known her a few hours. One night during my visit at about 1 o'clock in the morning, I went down to the kitchen to get a snack because I was hungry. Caroline happened to come in a few minutes after I sat down. She was roaring drunk and looking for a fight.

So she decided to amuse herself by talking to me. As she sat down, I could smell the stench of her drunkenness. She immediately began attacking me. "Who do you think you are? My family doesn't like you and neither do I!" She went on and on. I just thought to myself, "It's time for me to go." So as I was leaving she said, "You don't know anything about my family." Then she brought up the abuse issue. Obviously, it was a much bigger deal than I had thought with the whole of the family. Honestly, I wasn't aware that the "family" knew about it. At some point, the family had gone to great lengths to cover it up. I learned that it was in the news and such. Caroline made it clear whose side she was on. Her father never could have done something like that and her wretched sister was a liar. I really wasn't prepared for all this. So I left that conversation, only to find out in the morning that the spiteful sister went to her mother early in the morning, telling lies about me. I didn't realize it, but I had fallen into Caroline's trap. She was looking for anything to sabotage her sister's marriage. Suddenly, there was a great shift in the attitudes of both Amy's parents toward me.

Her father no longer approved of me and made it clear he did not approve of the marriage. The mother acted like I was the redheaded stepchild of the bunch. All of this emotional turmoil was very difficult for a three month sober twenty-year-old. Nevertheless, I stayed committed to our relationship even if her parents didn't approve. My family stepped up to the plate and told us that they would help us financially if we really wanted to be married. So we decided that I would move to Baton Rouge. When she entered college in the fall at LSU, I would enter junior college. I was prepared at this point, in the name of love, to leave my home state, family, sponsor, home-group, everything that I was accustomed to, in order to be with this woman.

After much deliberation and long sessions, I soothed the nerves of my parents. Assured that I could do well and stay clean, they supported my decision. My parents went above and beyond to ensure I had everything I would need. We found an apartment in Baton Rouge, completed the application, and eventually the day came—for me to move. I woke that morning at 4:30 a.m. and set out in my truck loaded down with everything I owned. It was a new day. I was so proud. I had journeyed from such a checkered past into manhood and responsibility. There aren't words to describe how I felt that day. I was so excited.

Inside of three hours, the truck broke down on Highway 20. After calling a towing service, they towed me to a garage. I waited and waited, eventually receiving the diagnosis that the water pump was shot. It took four hours for that repair, and then I was back on my way. I pulled into Baton Rouge that evening to start my new life. In the coming days, I would have all the amenities put in place: Television, internet, phone, so that I could work hard in school and become a husband. I went down and registered for college and it was done. I was ready to start my life.

Then the other shoe dropped. My fiancée, Amy, finally let her true colors come out. She cried most days from that time forward. Now that she had me, that wasn't enough. She was miserable all the time. Every day, we would endure her becoming more and more unhappy because

of her weight. She weighed one hundred and six pounds and stood 5'9".
Most girls would die to have a figure like hers. Yet she was consumed with
thoughts of how fat she was. Her emotions continued on a downward
trend and eventually she began talking about suicide. I felt very inad-
equate. Nothing I could do would please this girl. If it was sunny, she was
unhappy. If it was raining, she was despondent. This cycle grew worse as
the days passed. Before long, I had become resentful of her—the unrest
and depression was just too much. Days with her had seemed like being
trapped in a perpetual funeral of sobbing and weeping that had no end in
sight.

I started romancing the thought of escape. I thought if I could just
get rid of her when school starts, I could meet a normal girl. I just wanted
a way out, any way out. There had to be some relief from this misery. Soon,
the thought of using began its wretched nagging. I knew the thoughts
well. They were some of my most cherished memories and nightmares.
The thought of instant ecstasy filled the halls of my mind with excitement.
As each day grew more difficult, I would cling more to the pleasurable
memories of escape in using. One week before school started that year, I
had come to the end of my resolve. I left the apartment that morning in
search of what I knew would ease the pain—crack. Crack cocaine is ac-
cessible in every city in America. There is always somebody on some street
corner in the "wrong" part of town who will gladly show you where the
stuff is. It took me about 35 minutes to find it in Baton Rouge, a city I had
never used drugs in before.

I spent all day long slowly draining my bank account again. By the
evening, I was searching wildly for more money. You never think that using just once will set you on a path absolutely consumed with getting more
at any cost. That is exactly what happened to me every time I used. This
time was no different. Around 10 o'clock that evening, I stormed into the
apartment. I had just madly drunk a fifth of Crown Royal to ease the edge
of the crack. I sat down and confessed my use to Amy. She was distraught
and didn't know what to do. So while she called my mom, I went to the
room and got the rest of the cash I had. Then I left. The next thing I knew
I was coming to. When I resumed consciousness that evening I was in the
back of a DWI roadblock team's van. Police were finger printing me and
I was cussing and raising hell. All of the sudden I questioned why I was
under arrest. They informed me that I was jumping parking blocks in the
local grocery store parking lot in my truck! It must have been amusing
because I don't remember doing it.

Once I was bailed out of jail for the DWI, my mom, now in Baton Rouge, helped me pack everything up and take it back to Texas. Somehow in all the confusion, I convinced her to let me stay one more night with Amy and we would drive back to Texas together. She reluctantly agreed. My plot had worked. I still had a 5,000-dollar credit card in my pocket. Once the family was well on their way back to Texas, I headed to New Orleans. After I had "ruined" my opportunity, since the physical allergy had been awaked in me—now the obsession took control. So I disappeared for another three days in the heart of New Orleans with Amy's car. I sold everything but my shoes this time.

The only thing that stopped my crack binge this time was a car accident, which left me with my second DWI in three days. In jail again, this time in one of the worst city jails in America: Orleans parish. By this time, Amy's father, who hated me immensely, was hot on my trail. Since I had taken her car, he hunted me with a vengeance. Remember, he was a high-powered attorney in New Orleans. His means were endless and contacts sympathetic to his cause were numerous. He attempted to prevent me from having a bond set. He wanted to prosecute me beyond the law. In a place like New Orleans, having all his legal connections there, it was entirely possible.

This was a prominent, but by no means solitary, story of my own relapse—from my perspective. It started with recovery. I was working a program and staying clean. I was attempting to live a good life. My intentions were honorable and my heart was in the right place. Yet, I relapsed. Nothing "justifies" relapse. If a bad circumstance did, I would have been excused. Reality, family, and the legal system aren't that forgiving, though. The point in this chapter, from the annals of my life, is for you the reader to understand what relapse looks like. Now we ask the question: What was the cause of relapse? We now turn to analyze the facts so that we may determine some reasonable conclusions, which should help you in your recovery process.

Relapse happens when the commitment to stay clean and sober is broken. It was no mistake that I provided an extensive and compelling narrative about my relapse. You see, the details can mislead you from the most important truth. The reason my relapse and all relapse happens is that for one reason or another *the commitment to recovery and staying clean is broken.* No one uses, who does not first abandon their commitment to God, themselves, and their family to stay clean and sober. There are multitudes of perspectives from which you can peer, yet this truth remains foundational to them all. My narrative, like most addicts' stories, made using appear to be a viable, even logical option. My sickness convinced me that using was a solution to my problems. That called into question my commitment to recovery. When I reneged on my commitment, I was well on my way to relapse. No matter what "events, people, places, or things" occur, using is not an option. Regardless of the circumstance, *using is not an option.*

Relapse starts prior to the physical act of using. Most people would assume that relapse in my case started once I got to Baton Rouge, right? Wrong. Relapse in the above story started for me way back in Texas when I put a woman in front of my recovery. It happened when I became willing to leave my entire recovery network. Here my "relapse" started. This point cannot be stressed enough. While on staff at the House of Isaiah, many parents became focused on the circumstances of the actual use regarding their addict's relapse. That is to say, parents often assume in the case where two young men relapse together, the *other* addict is what made their loved one "fall off the wagon." That is simply not true. The focus needs to be directed to the beginning of relapse behavior, not the act of using. When you only kill the ants on the sidewalk, you never effectively treat the real problem, the nest underground. Relapse starts long before chemicals are used.

Relapse happens when recovery becomes secondary to anything of importance. Recovery is like taking medicine. When the patient takes the medicine it effects the illness—that is, the medicine does its job. The same is true with recovery, when the addict "takes their medicine" by going to meetings, praying, helping others, etc. then recovery is sustained. When this stops occurring, it may not happen immediately, but addiction begins to rear its head in the shadows. It quietly festers until it becomes a malignant tumor, multiplying in size and intensity. A recovering person must treat the illness or it will manifest itself. It is foolish for a sick patient, being weary, to stop taking his or her medicine. Addicts are no different. When something becomes more important than living sober (such as a job, girlfriend/wife, money, car, etc.), the addict is in *serious* trouble. If recovery takes second place to anything else in importance, relapse is at the door.

Does Relapse Happen to Everyone?

Regardless of what you're told, relapse does *not* happen to everyone. Relapse is *not* a part of recovery. The paradox, though, is that even though relapse is *not* a mandatory part of recovery, in many cases, it happens. Seldom does an addict get clean the first time and stay clean forever, although it does happen on occasion. I have found scores of parents and family members who are judgmental on the front end, when they encounter people who have relapsed. Usually, though, when the shoe is on the other foot, when the same thing befalls their loved one, it tends to have a humbling effect. Though you should *never expect* your loved one to relapse, you *should be aware and prepared* to deal with it if they do.

My mentor, Isiah Robertson, ingrained in my thinking, *"Proper Preparation Prevents Poor Performance."* This adage I live by and prescribe to everyone who will listen. Be prepared for anything, that way nothing catches you or your family off guard. The best kind of family is a prepared one. The family must be prepared to step in and make the right decisions if their loved one does relapse. Though it can be highly destructive, relapse doesn't mean defeat. No doubt, it is a setback in the big picture, but it lets you know your loved one has missed something vital in recovery and now they have the opportunity to face it and recover.

If your loved one doesn't resolve the true reason they relapsed, they will use again! As startling as this sounds, it really is true. Unresolved issues lead to eventual relapse if steps aren't taken to remedy the situation. Relapse (at very least) should be like an emergency warning light. When the light goes on, you know you've got problems. Even though the "car" didn't die on the side of the road, it's sure to down the road if you don't fix it. Whenever the addict relapses, make sure you address all the issues. Be exhaustive if necessary, no matter what the cost or the trouble. Find the reason or cause of the relapse and address it head on. This must be done so that the same thing doesn't happen again.

What Should I Do If My Loved One Relapses?

This is a question everyone affiliated with recovery should have an interest in. No one is "above" or "beyond" relapse. You, as the family of recovering persons, are responsible to be honest with yourself. The honest truth is that relapse can happen to the seemingly "best-case" in recovery. The question is: What will you do if your loved one relapses? The answer to that question can also mean the difference between life and death, freedom and prison. In my own story, you, the reader, were able to watch how much worse my "relapse" became, the longer I went without someone stopping me.

Relapse is bad. What is worse is when relapse goes un-addressed and the addict continues using, possibly racking up more legal charges, some of which they may not be able to overcome. This is a scenario no one expects, yet is possible with any addict. Some of the nicest people I've met went to prison because of their chemical dependency. These were not street bums, either. These men were insurance brokers, doctors, lawyers, and corporate executives. They were affluent, but that couldn't help them. Eventually, it doesn't matter how much money you have. When you get in enough trouble money can't even help you.

The way you can maximize your ability to assist the addict in your life and minimize the liability is to be prepared and have a plan. The plan should contain both choices and standards that will be held if relapse occurs. Also, whatever your plan is, make sure you are prepared emotionally to implement it. Plans are useless if you don't have the fortitude to carry them out.

What You Should Do If Your Loved One Relapses

1. *Stay calm*—As with any traumatic event, you must stay calm. Relapse most likely will be highly disappointing for you. Your feelings are important, but you must be rational. Do not allow your reaction to be emotionally driven as much as possible. Stay calm. The addict has engaged in using, so they have already excluded themselves from reasonable and rational thinking. You must not do the same.

2. *Assess the damage*—It is vital that you be aware of the warning signs. You may have even seen relapse coming, or you may be caught by surprise. Either way, you must be rational in assessing the damage. What you must do is ask many qualifying questions: Where? What? When? How? Be sure and probe the addict for any information they might not want to share out of shame, but that may be important. For instance, are the authorities looking for them? Have they committed any crimes to get the drugs? Is there anything they haven't told you?

3. *Damage control*—If your loved one is missing, do what you can to find them. If you cannot find them, be prepared to wait it out. They will turn up. Make sure your safety and their safety are taken care of. Remember, when they show up, you need to move quickly to get them to a safe and somewhat controlled environment. Damage control involves you absolving them of their car keys. That way, if they start feeling sad about

what they have done, they don't take the car in the middle of the night to go and use. You must remove any possible way they have of furthering their use. If that means taking their wallet, cash, credit cards, etc., *you do whatever is necessary.* You must be thorough—this is life or death and there are no second chances with the latter. Think through all possibilities and make sure you have secured your safety and theirs.

4. *Don't assume*—Never assume that a relapse is "just" a slip. While a relapse can be a slip, never assume anything. The addict has proved untrustworthy and now only *time* will aid this situation. Addicts who have used have ceased to be trustworthy for at least a few days. *Never assume that this relapse is over.* When you assume that everything will be just fine, you set your family up for more possible pain while endangering the addict. Remember: someone who is using illegal chemicals has already demonstrated the inability to use sound reasoning.

5. *Have a recovery plan*—This means have a concrete idea of what you will do if your loved one does relapse, in regard to getting them back on the right track. For instance, if your loved one relapses, you should be prepared to put them into a detoxification program if necessary. Also, it will be advisable to know what you will require of them, such as a certain amount of clean time before they can use their vehicle again. Remember, *no matter how old your loved one is*, if they are chemically dependent you must be willing to be the "parent/adult" in helping them get back on the right track.

6. *Be firm*—It is usually when addicts have acted their worst that they expect you to do what they want. They know the right things to say. It is your job not to be naive enough to accept "I promise, I'm really done this time." Everyone says that. If I've said it once, I've said that line a thousand times. The most common reaction of an addict's own relapse is to "down play" it. They will attempt to make the event out as if it were not such a big deal. The addict will always try any way possible to take the attention off of themselves. Be firm, because they will be exceptionally persuasive. The charming charisma flows when the fire is hot. *You must demand to see them live right, rather than make empty promises.*

7. *Follow through*—The most important thing an addict can learn is that when they use, *you will follow through.* They must know that using has consequences, even if they are not legal. Most chemically-dependent

persons seem to think if they're not in trouble with the law, their behavior isn't that bad. Wrong! You must follow through. If you say you will take away their car and stop financially supporting them, you must follow through. If you don't follow through, they will notice your weak behavior and take full advantage of you from that time forward.

8. *Finally, do not compromise*—Chemically-dependent persons' first instinct when their own behavior has backed them into a corner, is to play "Let's make a deal." Suddenly, now that they have used chemicals the addict has become willing to make a deal. If you demand they go to treatment, they will agree to do something, just not treatment. It's really amazing how addicted persons become such wonderful "attorneys," making all kinds of deals when *they are the ones without options*. You must assert that the addict's behavior and choices have removed their ability to make decisions for themselves and until they can show *over a period of time* that they have regained that ability—you, not them, should be making the decisions. Also, relapse puts *you*, now, in control whether you want to be or not. They will do what you demand, or they are welcome to go on down the road—that is the only way to reason with someone who has relapsed.

This is the test of your character. When and if your loved one relapses, it will be very trying for you. The biggest challenge for you will be whether you are able to stand up for the right thing even if it means them leaving. That is always the threat. When addicts in that condition have no other choice, they try and strike up a deal in order to assert some control again. Be prepared for them to threaten suicide. *Threats are normal.* Since they are "powerless" because of their choices, they will try various other ways of procuring relational influence. This can include, but is not limited to, a variety of threats. Here are some of the most common: threatening suicide, or physical harm to others, especially if you don't do what they want—not to mention threats that they will leave or kill themselves, etc. Many parents buckle under this type of pressure; I have personally witnessed it in my office. Always take threats seriously, but don't allow threats to *manipulate* you from doing the right thing.

The key in dealing with this problem is to render their threats powerless. How do you render their threats powerless? Simply assert that they have free will and they may choose to leave. They may choose to commit more crimes. They may choose anything they like. Just re-emphasize that no matter what they choose, you will not budge from your demands, and if they perpetuate negative behavior their life will be even more miserable. If you wait it out, they will think through it eventually. *Be prepared to let them go in the present to win them in the long run.* Even if they pack their bags then and there, don't budge. You must be willing to let them go if that's what it takes not to compromise. The same reason the U.S. Government refuses to negotiate with terrorists, you must *refuse* to negotiate with an addict that is using.

Doing the right thing is *not* always easy. If they do leave, you must be strong. Allow their own behavior to teach them. Once they realize life without your support is much more difficult than they thought, their attitude will change. In this case, when they do come back, there will be a certain willingness to do what is asked of them. This can save their life. In my experience, I have seen more than one young man die unnecessarily because his parents didn't have the backbone to stand firm. The parents were scared and their own fear permitted the addict in the situation to continue making his own decisions. Those families don't have a second chance to stand up for what is right. Their children died chemically dependent. Don't let your children/loved one(s) die; lift up a standard and stick with it, at all costs.

Conclusion

This chapter should have provided you extensively with a *guide* to understand and protect yourself from relapse. Relapse doesn't happen to everyone, but it does happen to some. Expect the best and be prepared for the worst. Your loved one is an investment in human life. You have an interest in them; protect it like you would any investment.

If your loved one is in recovery you should be, too. Never think yourself exempt from recovery. If they have a support network you should, too. There are many options for families to get the support they need. Al-Anon is a wonderful program to support the families of alcoholics and addicts. You should have a network of individuals for support so that if something happens with your loved one, you have the support necessary to help them the best that you can. Armed with these tools, you will be empowered to stand up to the pressures of an addict who relapses and help them to—*Recover All!*

14

Top Ten Issues to Avoid

THROUGH MY experience working at the House of Isaiah, I have worked with hundreds of addicts and their families. During that time I have seen many addicts recover and many fail to recover. Some have begun their lives anew, going out from the program, rebuilding their lives, and becoming productive members of society. Others went back to using. Of the latter many went to prisons and tragically some even lost their lives. While in the final analysis it is the addict that must experience the psychic change from within to successfully recover from addiction, there is an element of involvement in which the family takes part. There are behaviors that family members can practice which are conducive to recovery. Conversely, there are some actions family members can exhibit that have dire consequences upon the addict. Below I have assimilated what I hold to be the ten things that, in my experience, proved the worst and sadly most common practices/behaviors family members took part in that were detrimental to the addict's recovery process. It would be incredulous to think that these were the *only* ten; they are not. However, these are some of the most common and are offered for your benefit to guard you against the mistakes others before you have made.

10. Don't break the anonymity of your loved one.

When a person embarks on the wondrous journey we call recovery, it is very hard. There are a lot of adjustments that must be made. It is in the family's best interest to be as supportive as possible, both for the individual health of their loved one and also their ability to function in the family unit. A sensitive area for many addicts/alcoholics is their anonymity. Anonymity is a term used to convey the practice of being anonymous with reference to something. Usually, your loved one will learn about anonymity in the arena of Alcoholics/Narcotics Anonymous meetings. One reason the group calls themselves "Alcoholics Anonymous" is because it is their aim to provide a safe atmosphere for anyone to share within the group. Outside of the meetings, it would be inappropriate for a member of A.A.

to address another member in public about A.A. or alcoholism. Their recovery program is anonymous, unless they so choose to share with others about their participation.

You might be thinking at this point, "If the addict doesn't tell people around them about their addiction how can they stay sober?" First, the addict chooses to stay sober, others cannot do that for them. Secondly, it is each individual's responsibility to go places and associate with people conducive to their recovery. The problem most family members make with anonymity is best described by way of an illustration. For instance, let's say my mother and I were out at a restaurant with family and friends. It happens to be someone in the group's birthday, so many people are celebrating and some people in the group are drinking. My mother and I are sitting next to each other and when the waitress comes around to take our drink orders, the friend next to me asks if I want a beer. It's a simple question. They don't know I attend A.A. or that I'm recovering from alcoholism. Well, before I can open my mouth—my mother spurts out, "No, he *can't* have a beer, he's in recovery."

Now you might be thinking that's a little over-protective. What's the big deal, right? First of all, my recovery is not the business of the waitress or my friend unless I choose for it to be. Secondly, I have just been publicly humiliated because of my recovery. Now people think they have to watch their drinks around me. You never know, I might slip off the wagon and chug all the beer on the table while the birthday-boy blows out candles! Sure, this is exaggerated for effect. Nevertheless, anonymity was so important to the founders of A.A. and its beginning that they included anonymous in the name as well as making the twelfth tradition read, "Anonymity is the spiritual foundation of all our Traditions, ever reminding us to place principles before personalities."[1] Especially in early recovery, always realize some people are shy about their recovery, some more than others. It is their right to be. As the family, you're responsible to support them, not to alert others to their sobriety!

9. Don't fall into the emotional trap of being jealous of your loved one's new lifestyle and friends in recovery.

In the early days of your loved one's recovery, they will probably become enthralled with the A.A./N.A. program. Remember using chemicals was more than just a behavior. It was a lifestyle. Part of why the A.A./N.A. program is so successful is because each group has multitudes of activities

1. "The Twelve Traditions," available at http://www.aa.org/bigbookonline/en_appendiceI. cfm; accessed 19 May 2007.

and fellowship to be involved in. It is essential that your loved one develop friend-relationships with other people in recovery. These people will form their support network. They will also be instrumental in the long-term sobriety of your loved one. Many times, these new friends and activities capture a great deal of the newly recovering addict's time and attention. Sometimes family members feel neglected during this time.

It can even seem at times that the newly recovering person has lost interest in home and family for their new recovery lifestyle. The family, in turn, often feels that they have endured the tragic times of active addiction and *now* the addict has the audacity to pay attention to everyone except the family who stuck by their side. If you feel this way, understand that your feelings are valid. Furthermore, you are not alone in these feelings. That fact alone doesn't remedy the situation, but realize that this is an important phase in the recovery of your loved one. You may need to express in a non-confrontational way your feelings. You might need to seek private professional counseling (with the addict) in order to communicate effectively what you are experiencing and what your needs are. Keep in mind, this process is normal. It is vital that you not allow yourself to become jealous because eventually jealousy breeds resentment.

If you become jealous and resentful of the very program and friends your loved one is using to stay clean and sober, this really puts the addict in a tough spot. The essential thing to remember is that *you need to be in recovery as well*. Addiction affects the whole family. Even if you think you don't have a problem, you need to be in a support group for families of the addicted (Al-Anon®) or something similar. If you participate in a support group that offers you a variety of social activities and opportunities to develop new friendships, both you and the addict will be developing together your own social support networks. Indeed, the only successful way to combat becoming jealous is for you to work a program of recovery. Indeed, some family members struggle with the idea of them needing to "work a program." Virtually all humans, for some reason, resist change. It is often thought, "they [the addict] has the problem, why do I have to change . . . ?" Yet there is still emotional healing that must take place in your heart from all the damage that has been done during the course of your loved one's addiction. Take this challenge directly, be encouraged in your own growth and take steps not to become jealous of the addict's new found life in recovery.

8. Don't assume the addict knows the rules and the boundaries you have; reiterate and make clear what you require.

It's easy to assume that your loved one is fully aware of what you require with regards to rules and/or boundaries. You should explain your rules, that is, if they live in your house subsequent to treatment or if they come home on pass from a treatment program, let them know what you expect. Regardless of whether they lived with you before and *you expect* that they already know the rules—odds are you should tell them again. Pretend as though you are dealing with a brand new family member that you've never met before who will be staying in your house. There is little doubt that you expect them to know coming home at two or three in the morning is unacceptable. However, frequently addicts exhibit a strange phenomenon in early recovery—"isolated amnesia." People early in recovery typically suppose that since they are no longer using drugs or alcohol that they can do whatever they desire. Furthermore, I have known many parents who, after confronting their recovering person with misbehavior hear the reply, "But I wasn't using!" Don't be one of those, prepare ahead, articulate your expectations that way everyone involved understands.

We should also caution you regarding the establishment of rules. We find that within family/addict relations there exists four types of relationships in regard to the establishment of rules or boundaries. These types describe in broad spectrum the overall relationship between addict and family in regard to expectations or rules: undefined, extreme, unpredictable, and clear rules. The situation in which we find undefined rules is in the scenario of silence. This occurs when no expectation is expressed specifically. Therefore, if you expect the addict home by 11 p.m. during the week, but you don't say that explicitly. This is unhealthy for both parties. The addict doesn't have a clear idea of what they ought to do and the family has failed to communicate. Thus, when the addict comes home at twelve, the family scolds him or her for breaking the rules. This scenario becomes very frustrating for all parties involved. You should be clear about what you expect, no matter what it is. That way the addict has a clear understanding of what behavior is acceptable and what is not. Undefined rules are inconsistent.

Secondly, we have the scenario of extreme rules. This situation occurs where the family sets unreasonably high expectations. Usually this takes place by the family member who has been hurt by the addict. Sometimes the family member does this in order to "help" keep the addict "in line." Either way, this scenario, in an effort to have a strong defense, creates dissention. The addict becomes resentful by overburdening load of new responsibilities coupled with staying sober, which makes for an unhappy person to be around. This dynamic starts a process of driving both addict and family apart from each another. And thus, it is detrimental to all involved. The goal is for the family *not* to enable the addict, but also *not to disable* them. There must be a harmony found between the extremes.

Thirdly, we have the case of unpredictable rules. This happens when the family keeps "upping the ante"—so to speak. Sometimes when addict begins to do well, the family starts increasing the requirements. If done in a very slow systematic way, this can actually be helpful. However, in most cases where this occurs it is neither done in a slow nor systematic fashion. This leaves the person in recovery constantly unable to satisfy the demands. No one, whether addicted or not, enjoys living in an environment with people whose expectations are changing everyday. In early recovery, addicts need consistency. The family has the ability to assist in this by providing a relational atmosphere of communication of needs, feelings, and especially expectations. Again, *balance* can't be emphasized enough, it is vital.

Finally, we have the healthy scenario of clear rules. In this circumstance there are clear rules that give broad boundaries to the relationship for all the parties involved. These are firm, though not excessive, rules. This is a safe balance between undefined and extreme as well as unpredictable rules. Balance provides an atmosphere were all parties have optimal opportunity to be emotionally healthy.

For you to have healthy rules, you must be clear about what is and is not acceptable behavior. An example of this could be seen in a family who makes boundaries which are both safe and reasonable for the individual. For instance, a family gives the recovering person some freedoms while maintaining a reasonable and safe system of structure. We want to give them rope, just not enough to hang themselves. It is the responsibility of the family to uphold boundaries and be firm in them. Jeremy's story is a good example. He was a 24-year-old man who was living with his parents prior to his inpatient treatment, from which, he had just graduated. Therefore, having successfully completed long-term inpatient treatment, he wanted to return home to establish his life again, begin working and saving money in order to move out on his own.

However, his parents made the responsible decision to *require* him to continue his recovery in a halfway home which provided a more structured environment than at home. He will now have many freedoms that he was not allowed while inpatient. Further, he will be expected to find gainful employment while attending both A.A. and church meetings. His parents agreed, at first, to assist Jeremy financially so he would have a good start. In doing this they covered his first month's rent at the halfway home, enabling him the opportunity to find a job. Also, they agreed to provide him with fifty dollars a week so he would be able to buy some groceries and have gas to get to his interviews. Part of Jeremy's problem—other than drugs—was his financial dependence upon his family.

The first few weeks went by and Jeremy didn't find a job, though he affirmed that he had been looking for work and submitting applications. During this time, he called his mother numerous times in despair. He told her of his great need for more money. Of course, she questioned him and told him clearly that he better get his spending under control because she was not going to just give him money all the time. Begrudgingly, she still gave him the money every week. As more time passed Jeremy still hasn't found a job. Nevertheless, the weekly routine continued of begging for money. Finally, some of the staff confronted Jeremy's mother about her enabling. But she wasn't able to tell him no. He would beg and plead, ultimately getting his way. Since Jeremy was sustaining his financial need through his parents, he didn't find a job because he really didn't want to; sure he filled out applications, but he wasn't serious about finding one. What is more, he has no reason to. Why would he get a job when his finances are taken care of? Sure, he has to endure lectures and a little scolding, but what he was doing worked. Why should he change?

Here is an example of unhealthy rules/boundaries. This most accurately depicts undefined boundaries because even though she had stated her "boundary" of how much money she would give, continually she proved that when that boundary is crossed, she would back up and draw another line! That negates the entire principle of having a rule or boundary. It should be obvious that the above four distinctions extend beyond the mere concept of a "rule," for instance, simply to come home at a certain time. This extends to *how and what* you will do in order to assist the addict. So each week, the mother's boundary changed to fit the situation. The line wasn't clearly drawn. Hence, this was an undefined boundary. It prevented the emotional growth and maturity of Jeremy. Again, you might be thinking, "I would never allow my kid to walk all over me like that!" It is always easier to say when it's not your kid. The reality is when it *is* your loved one, it becomes much more difficult to clearly distinguish. So as responsible parents and family members, don't assume they know your rules and boundaries reiterate and make them crystal-clear.

7. Allow your loved one to be responsible for their own responsibilities.

Active addiction can debilitate the addict's ability and desire to handle their own responsibilities. Often this is reflected in a lazy attitude toward promptly taking care of personal responsibilities. Usually the family, during the course of addiction, will begin assuming certain responsibilities such as medical appointments, probationary responsibilities, and other responsibilities. This often happens prior to the addict getting into treatment because that is the time at which typically the greatest chaos has ensued. While the addict is in treatment often the family takes off the "slack" and handles certain responsibilities for them. A problem that arises is that subsequent to the addict graduating from the treatment program, either: 1) the addict fails to take responsibilities for these tasks, or 2) the family is reluctant to turn these responsibilities back over to them. Either way, this behavior is destructive in the long-term. The addict *must* assume responsibility for themselves, the health of their recovery process could very well hinge on it.

A few examples here will help us to fully realize the potential downfall this could cause for your loved one. First, let me introduce you to Tommy. Tommy completed inpatient treatment. Part of Tommy's past includes some extensive legal problems, which left him with a number of probationary responsibilities. This required him to attend specific meetings, classes, and appointments to satisfy the court. These meetings were above and beyond A.A. and any other activity he would need to do to maintain his personal recovery program. Tommy's mother, while he was in treatment, had been keeping up with his many appointments. Indeed, she had a special planner just to keep track of the responsibilities. She was scrupulous in detail because Tommy's freedom lay in balance. However, after Tommy left treatment, she continued to maintain his appointments. This was problematic for a number of reasons. First, Tommy became resentful because he felt she always "controlled" and dictated his actions, not to mention the perceived nagging he had grown to hate. Thus, it drove them apart. Also, Tommy never developed the necessary confidence and self-respect one naturally gets from being responsible.

After some time, even Tommy started fighting her to let go of managing the tasks. His mother was genuinely afraid, namely, that Tommy wasn't going to manage the tasks properly and ultimately get sent back to prison. Her concern was, of course, warranted. Yet it was preventing Tommy from growing. Tommy should have been solely responsible, at the age of 24, with some clean time under his belt to meet all his requirements. His mother meant well, and her heart was right. But the responsibility is Tommy's. Until she let go, he couldn't grow. The probationary requirements were Tommy's. The longer his mother managed them the longer Tommy was forced to be dependent. This was counter-productive. Even if Tommy did forget an appointment, he should have had to learn to bear the responsibility and burden of consequence. Now this illustration can be used in any similar situation, not just in the case of probation. I've seen cases over having extensive dentist surgery or any number of other responsibilities. Allow the recovering person to slowly, but surely regain all of his or her own personal responsibility. This will benefit all parties involved.

6. Do not work their program for them.

This advice builds upon the previous error. It can be very easy for a family member to begin working their loved one's program. What we mean here is that a mother or wife can become so involved with making sure the loved one is doing everything they should be doing to stay sober, such as attending meetings, calling their sponsor etc., that it takes away the responsibility of the individual. This time we will look at the experience of Jim. Jim was a 37-year-old husband and father. He had just completed inpatient treatment. Upon moving home, his former employer allowed him to return to work. Things seemed to fall right into place. His wife, Jill, had been extremely supportive of his recovery. During the entire ordeal she stood by his side, was very forgiving, and was extensively involved in recovery herself. She really wanted to be the best wife she could be to her husband for both of their recovery.

She had attended Al-Anon and had set up boundaries. Every recommendation that the treatment center and counselors had for her, she did. She was very compliant and eager to learn. So when Jim did finally move home, she was well aware of what it meant to work a quality recovery program. Since she had all this knowledge and was eager to help her husband, she would always ask him if he went to his meetings. She became his "watchdog." She feared so greatly that Jim would fall back into active addiction that she was willing to work very hard to ensure his sobriety. A man really couldn't ask for a better partner in Jim's situation. It became a daily thing for her to run through her checklist for him. "Did you pray? Good. Did you go to your meeting? Good. Did you call your sponsor? Good." On and on down the list she would go. Surely you can tell that this took all the responsibility off Jim. Not only did it aggravate him, it also caused unneeded tension and distance between them.

Jim felt that she didn't have any confidence in his ability to stay clean and sober. Jill was just scared that Jim would relapse. Both parties had good intentions. Jill, however, could not work Jim's program, and yet that was just what she was doing. What Jim needed was to be responsible to take care of his recovery. Caution should be exercised here in order to be clear, namely, if Jim was *not* working a program, then Jill attempting to hold him accountable would be perfectly acceptable. However, in this case, Jill was attempting to work his program *for him*. Even if it means failure and sometimes relapse, the addict must be responsible for their own recovery, or it won't last. As we have stated previously, you are unable to keep the addict clean and sober. Even if you quit work and stayed home to guard them twenty-four hours a day, you still couldn't, inevitably, prevent them from using. Do *not* work your loved one's program. It hurts them. It hurts you. It hurts your relationship.

5. Realize your loved one doesn't always tell you the truth.

To the average person, this might seem like a give in. Yet this is a huge trap families fall into, especially while their loved one is in an inpatient program. What happens is the addict plays a game. The game is about manipulation. The game is to get desired results. This game involves pulling the right strings on each puppet to manipulate them around on the stage in order to bring the "show" to an expected end. Here I will use my own life as the specimen. I was notorious for telling half-truths to get people to do things (of course, others weren't aware of this). I was methodical, precise, and very, very convincing. Let me share with you the techniques I used to get what I wanted. I will share these in order to illuminate the devices and tactics of good-hearted people who are sick with addiction.

My mother and I have always had a very open relationship when it comes to communication. I have generally always told her the truth (at least she thought), except in the case of drugs and alcohol. This became the chief and most strategic way of me furthering my manipulation once I ceased using chemicals. Remember, being dry (no chemicals) does not mean being in recovery. While abstinence is the foundation of recovery, it alone does not constitute recovery. With that said, during the course of my treatment, as with most addicts/alcoholics in early recovery, I was focused on everything outside of myself. My attention was fixated on the staff of the treatment program and what they were doing. Also, my focus was on the other clients and what they were doing. Mostly I focused on everything wrong. I was obsessed with practices I considered ridiculous or irrational.

What you need to understand is that *I was building a case*. Each time I communicated with my mom on the phone or at visitation, I would always give her the latest gossip about what was going on at the treatment program. I would give her the run down of how the staff acted irrationally, or how the director (in my opinion) didn't handle another client's issues correctly, or who had snuck drugs on the property and relapsed. Slowly, day-by-day, week-by-week, I was building a case and building influence with my family. It was so subtle that no one noticed. What I did was espionage. Systematically, I began doing everything in my power to erode the credibility of the treatment program I was in. I did this by only shedding partial light on a subject. For instance, when I would tell my mom the events, I would only present one side. Anyone from the outside looking in could figure out that was biased.

So after a period of time, I had accumulated and transmitted enough one-sided information that I had actually called into question, at least in my mother's mind, the credibility and ability of the staff at the treatment program I was a patient in. Sounds devious; it is. Don't put it past your loved one, sometimes this behavior even becomes second nature to the addict. Certainly, I'm not asserting that all recovering persons are liars, but they are *masters* at casting light on a topic in such a way as to only illuminate specific areas to influence the choices of others. All addicts/alcoholics are able to exhibit this behavior, it simply comes with the territory. Therefore, you must make the choice to trust in those staff members at the treatment program that you select for your addict to get help. *They are professionals* and while they may not always do things you understand or even agree with, they do know what they are doing.

I would never argue that you should keep your addict in a program that endangers their well-being. However, I have seen many family members make poor decisions to allow their addict to leave treatment, on the basis of being manipulated by the addict—usually in regard to the treatment center or staff. Remember, the addict attempts to divert attention from their behavior and progress in order to manipulate circumstances.

4. Secrets keep you sick; you are not responsible to keep their secrets.

This truth is applicable regardless of circumstance. Secrets keep people sick. The more secrets your loved one has that they refuse to be honest about, the longer they will stay emotionally unhealthy. Keeping secrets means consciously withholding information. It is never healthy to keep secrets. Addicts and alcoholics are professionals at playing the secret game. The secret game is the practice of keeping certain secrets from certain people. Underneath the innocent looking surface is the fundamental problem: deception. The longer people in recovery keep secrets, the longer they are held in bondage to those secrets. Working a recovery program means "coming clean" and letting go of secrets.

There is great power in telling the truth. Here is an example of the way most secrets are initiated and kept occur along these lines. Suppose Freddie got in trouble at school. The teacher called his home and informed his mother of the behavior he had expressed. When Freddie came home from school, she confronted him about his inappropriate behavior at school. However, in an effort to keep the home in peace for the evening she conceded *not to tell his dad this time*. But if Freddie did it again, she would surely tell him. The problem is this: any time we keep something from another person, we are keeping a secret. To intentionally overlook a circumstance is to initiate a secret and essentially lie. Even though it seems harmless for the sake of having a nice evening—not to tell Dad, it gives Freddie the idea that there are things Mom can and will keep from Dad.

Now if Freddie is really clever, he will figure out the converse is probably also true—that there are some things Dad might keep from Mom under given circumstances. So what does Freddie do? He plays both sides against the middle, effectively controlling the whole of the family units' relationships with deception and secrets. Whenever people keep secrets, they are forced to behave accordingly. Eventually, steps must be taken somewhere down the road to insure the confidentiality of the secret. Sometimes lies have to "cover" for other lies. It can really do great damage to any attempted recovery program. How do you stop the process of secrets? Don't allow your loved one to tell you a secret. What we mean is that when they ask you not to tell, it will only take one time to get your point across. You make clear that you will in *no* way participate in *not telling* anything to anyone. Once the addict knows you are serious, their weaponry of manipulation will be disabled. You can stop this sickness dead in its tracks if you are informed and prepared.

3. Don't participate in the guilt game.

Another thing that families can especially be detoured by is the infliction of guilt in the relationship. Addicts who find themselves in treatment are powerless. They are powerless over their lives, in that, they have ceased to be in control of their own lives on a daily basis. Furthermore, in an attempt to "win back" some type of influence or control the addict becomes willing to do virtually anything. Employing guilt as a tool to win influence in a relationship is one tactic. We have dealt elsewhere with guilt, here we are primarily concerned with a few possible situations. Are you aware that guilt can be used against you in an attempt to control you? It could manifest by means of the addict attempting get money from you or in order for you to do something they want. Thus, guilt is used to cause an effect that is pleasant to the recovering person.

Your goal should be to recognize that the past is the past. That is to say, what is done is done. Guilt only works on those who can be manipulated into focusing on the past in such a way that it influences their decisions in the present. No one, especially in the case of addiction, has acted perfectly or always said the "right" things. Regardless of harsh words you have spoken in difficult situations or poor decisions, looking back you would have made differently, the past is done. Keeping this in mind will help you prevent from being manipulated through guilt. Even if you're loved one blames their drug use on you or says, "If you would have . . ." The proper response is to calmly and clearly tell the addict that you are not responsible neither for their behavior nor their feelings. Your loved one used drugs and alcohol because *they chose to*. Addicts tend to come up with many reasons to blame others for their own problems. At the end of the day, however, they bear the responsibility. The addict is the one who puts the drugs into their bodies and chooses to break the law, acting foolishly. No matter what you have done, they have to be responsible for their own actions, not you. *Deny your loved one the ability to make you feel guilty.* You may have done things wrongly, even horribly wrong, but giving in to their manipulation won't change that.

2. Don't fall in the other ditch; they can't be blamed for everything.

While you cannot allow your loved one to "eat your lunch" by trying to inflict guilt, you must be cautious not to blame everything on them. Since the addict has caused so much destruction due to their active using, it can be all too easy for them to become the scapegoat. No doubt, the addict may have caused exceedingly unpleasant circumstances to befall you or your family. Just as the addict using guilt to manipulate you is detrimental, so also is it hurtful for the family to perpetually blame circumstances on the addict. That is, when one creates an environment for the addict in which they frequently feel attacked or as though their role is that of the "scapegoat" virtually no one can be happy. No one likes to be constantly reminded of their past mistakes. Therefore, a significant attempt should be made continually to do the emotional work necessary to heal from past hurts. Forgiveness is tough to practice, yet it is necessary for the health of all in a relationship. Thus, whatever "baggage" you may be carrying as a result of the addict's behavior or addiction needs to be dealt with in a healthy way. If you are unsure or find yourself incapable of pursuing forgiveness in this way, we suggest you seek professional counseling. Not to mention that if you are constantly pointing the finger, it won't be long before the addict develops an attitude of indifference. This might manifest in the "everybody is against me" mentality. This behavior is more common in marriage relationships. Be proactive, be healthy, and do not blame others.

1. You can't fix them.

Sometimes the hardest thing to accept is that you can't fix the addict. No doubt, it is always sad when a parent or family member desires the recovery of the addict more than they do. The harsh reality remains that no matter how much you want it for them, you can't fix them. The ability doesn't lie within you to cause them to get better and neither can you give them the desire to say sober. *Recovery is not possible unless the addict's desire to stay clean becomes greater than their desire to use.* We don't have power over others' desires. We are unable to impart desire into others. Certainly, we can encourage and exhort, even at times resorting to "strongly advising" and other tactics of getting through to them. At the end of the day, though, we can't fix them.

For instance, Jeff was a brilliant twenty-two-year-old young man. He came from a very wealthy family and had been educated at the finest schools. From the outside, one would think that this individual had every good opportunity anyone could want. The only problem was that Jeff was an alcoholic, a real alcoholic. The *Alcoholics Anonymous* text's description fit him precisely. He had the matchless ability to get stark raving drunk at the most inopportune times. As a result, he caused his affluent family a great deal of social disdain with his insane behavior. Even worse than that, he was driving his parents crazy. He demanded their attention at all times of the day and night. There was always some chaotic dilemma he found himself in the middle of.

His parents finally brought him to treatment. He was more than a handful. Regardless of all the helpful people, counseling, and program, he was determined not to get sober. Under no uncertain terms would he cease from drinking. No one could convince him. He learned to play the treatment game. He said the right things to appease the staff and his family. It was obvious he didn't mean any of it. We dealt with him in and out of treatment for over sixteen months. Today he stays drunk around the clock. Sometimes he even calls the treatment center completely intoxicated just to amuse himself. He has no desire to get sober. His parents spent a fortune. They would have given anything just for their son to be sober. They couldn't fix him. Neither could the treatment staff. He will remain drunk until is desire to be sober exceeds his desire to remain in misery. You must resolve within yourself that no matter what happens with your loved one, you will be okay. You can do your best, but you can do no more. You can't fix them, as much as you would like to try. *Acceptance is the first step towards recovery.* The addict is powerless over alcohol and drugs. Conversely, you are powerless over them.

Conclusion

These ten principles should help you in aiding in your loved one's recovery. Sometimes the best offense is a good defense. The more you are aware of your own behavior and consciously think about the solution, the more opportunity you have to succeed. Recovery is a long process. It doesn't happen over night. In my own life, it took years of heartache before a glimmer of light shined through the darkness. Never lose heart and never quit believing. If God did it for me, he can do it for you. Stay aware of these ten issues and your family will be well on their way to—*Recover All!*

15

Conclusion

IT IS my earnest prayer that through the experience and practical wisdom shared in this work you have been equipped to better understand and face whatever addictive problems may come against your family. Addiction, of any kind, is not a simple illness with a quick and easy remedy. However, when empowered with understanding and faith that *it can* get better you should be able to face the opposition head-on and achieve victory. The hardest thing to do when faced with a loved one's addiction is not to give up. You have encountered numerous examples of what not to do. Now the responsibility rests on you to be the strong family member who is both wise and loving in assisting them to recover from a hopeless state of mind and body. Those who press into the power of God and stand against the wiles of addictive scheming will *Recover All!*

Bibliography

Alcoholics Anonymous. Fourth edition. New York: Alcoholics Anonymous World Services, 2001.

Bauer, Walter. *A Greek-English Lexicon of the New Testament and Other Early Christian Literature.* Revised and Edited by Frederick Danker. 3d Edition. Chicago: University of Chicago, 2000.

Lenski, R.C.H. *The Interpretation of St. Paul's First and Second Epistle to the Corinthians.* Minneapolis, MN: Augsburg, 1963.

Silkworth, William D. "The Doctor's Opinion." In *Alcoholics Anonymous.* Fourth edition. New York: Alcoholics Anonymous World Services, 2001.

Wink, Walter. *Naming the Powers: The Language of Power in the New Testament. The Powers: Volume 1.* 3 Vols. Philadelphia: Fortress Press, 1984.